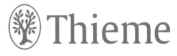

Neurological Diseases

Implications in Medical and Dental Practices

Armin Ariana, MMed, MD, PhD
Senior Lecturer in Medical Education
Course Convenor, General Pathology
The School of Medicine and Dentistry
Griffith University
Griffith Health Centre
Queensland, Australia

Contributor:
Haleh Vosgha, PhD
Post-Doctoral Research Fellow
The School of Medicine
Griffith University
Griffith Health Centre
Queensland, Australia

25 illustrations

Thieme
New York • Stuttgart • Delhi • Rio de Janeiro

Library of Congress Cataloging-in-Publication Data

Names: Ariana, Armin, author.

Title: Neurological diseases : implications in medical and dental practices / Armin Ariana.

Description: New York : Thieme Medical Publishers, Inc., [2020] | Includes bibliographical references and index.

Identifiers: LCCN 2019027185| ISBN 9781684202249 (paperback) | ISBN 9781684202270 (ebook)

Subjects: | MESH: Nervous System Diseases–diagnosis | Nervous System Diseases–therapy | Patient Care | Dental Care for Chronically Ill

Classification: LCC RC346 | NLM WL 140 | DDC 616.8–dc23 LC record available at https://lccn.loc.gov/2019027185

Copyright © 2020 by Thieme Medical Publishers, Inc.

Thieme Publishers New York
333 Seventh Avenue, New York, NY 10001 USA
+1 800 782 3488, customerservice@thieme.com

Thieme Publishers Stuttgart
Rüdigerstrasse 14, 70469 Stuttgart, Germany
+49 [0]711 8931 421, customerservice@thieme.de

Thieme Publishers Delhi
A-12, Second Floor, Sector-2, Noida-201301
Uttar Pradesh, India
+91 120 45 566 00, customerservice@thieme.in

Thieme Revinter Publicações Ltda.
Rua do Matoso, 170 – Tijuca
Rio de Janeiro RJ 20270-135 - Brasil
+55 21 2563-9702
www.thiemerevinter.com.br

Cover design: Thieme Publishing Group
Typesetting by Thomson Digital, India

Printed in the United States of America by King Printing Co., Inc.   5 4 3 2 1

ISBN 978-1-68420-224-9

Also available as an e-book:
eISBN 978-1-68420-227-0

Important note: Medicine is an ever-changing science undergoing continual development. Research and clinical experience are continually expanding our knowledge, in particular our knowledge of proper treatment and drug therapy. Insofar as this book mentions any dosage or application, readers may rest assured that the authors, editors, and publishers have made every effort to ensure that such references are in accordance with **the state of knowledge at the time of production of the book.**

Nevertheless, this does not involve, imply, or express any guarantee or responsibility on the part of the publishers in respect to any dosage instructions and forms of applications stated in the book. **Every user is requested to examine carefully** the manufacturers' leaflets accompanying each drug and to check, if necessary in consultation with a physician or specialist, whether the dosage schedules mentioned therein or the contraindications stated by the manufacturers differ from the statements made in the present book. Such examination is particularly important with drugs that are either rarely used or have been newly released on the market. Every dosage schedule or every form of application used is entirely at the user's own risk and responsibility. The authors and publishers request every user to report to the publishers any discrepancies or inaccuracies noticed. If errors in this work are found after publication, errata will be posted at www.thieme.com on the product description page.

Some of the product names, patents, and registered designs referred to in this book are in fact registered trademarks or proprietary names even though specific reference to this fact is not always made in the text. Therefore, the appearance of a name without designation as proprietary is not to be construed as a representation by the publisher that it is in the public domain.

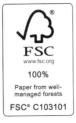

This book is dedicated to all junior practitioners who are about to help their patients with neurological diseases.

It is also in memory of those who have struggled with ALS.

Contents

1 Introduction

Armin Ariana

Neurological and neurodegenerative diseases have significant effects on functionality, independency, and overall quality of life of a patient. As the degenerative progression manifests throughout the course of these diseases, patients develop more severe symptoms, and as a consequence, many aspects of the patients' health are compromised. Unfortunately, in spite of the advance of contemporary medical technology, these diseases are, still, incurable, and none of the treatments available can slow down the degenerative process.[1]

Researchers have been focusing on achieving a deeper understanding of the mechanisms and processes of these neurological diseases and on advancing imaging techniques such as MRI. Despite ongoing research, the causes of most of these conditions are not completely known, and their pathophysiology remains poorly understood.

Parkinson disease, for example, is a chronic neuropathological disorder involving progressive degeneration of dopaminergic and non-dopaminergic neurons present in the substantia nigra.[2] This neuronal degenerative activity causes a loss of voluntary motor control, and patients develop characteristic motor symptoms.[2,3]

Multiple sclerosis (MS) is another example of a chronic autoimmune disease that affects the central nervous system (CNS), and it is characterized by the inflammation, demyelination, and scarring (sclerosis: Greek for scarring) of nerve tissues.[4,5,6] It is the most common cause of neurological disability in young adults[7] with an overall increasing prevalence worldwide regardless of age.[8]

Amyotrophic lateral sclerosis (ALS), the most common fatal neurodegenerative disease, is another example of a progressive disorder in this series.[9] ALS is a non-cell-autonomous disease that targets the motor neurons and the surrounding glia.[10]

Alzheimer disease (AD) is known as the common cause of dementia, with its insidious onset causing the progressive impairment of memory and other cognitive functions. Alzheimer's diagnosis relies primarily on the mental decline, with no motor, sensory, or coordination problems evident in the early stages. AD is a progressive, degenerative brain disease, and it affects up to 70% of people that suffer from dementia, with an estimated 115.4 million people predicted as sufferers by the year 2050.[11] Its incidence and prevalence is linked to the increase in age.[12]

This book then reviews "Stroke," which, despite being a preventable and treatable disease, has become a global epidemic of the 21st century. In 2010, an estimated 16.9 million stroke incidents occurred, of which 5.9 million lives were lost; this makes stroke the second leading cause of death after ischemic heart disease.[13] Caused by an inadequate blood supply to the brain, cerebrovascular accident or stroke can potentially lead to functional impairments, severe brain damage, and, consequently, death.[14] Common long-term effects include contralateral limb paralysis, memory loss, and cognitive impairment.[14]

Epilepsy is one of the most prevalent neurological disorders presenting with recurrent episodes of seizures, affecting an estimated 50 million individuals worldwide. They are regarded as a collection of conditions with different pathophysiologies, multiple manifestations, and diverse aetiologies.[15] It is caused by the abnormal electrical activity of the brain, specifically, uncontrolled discharges from groups of neurons—hyperexcitability of the neurons of the cerebral hemispheres.[16] Epilepsy is a disorder that can present at all ages, affecting both males and females, with males at a slightly higher risk.[16] Due to lack of consciousness following an epileptic attack, patients may seriously injure themselves, potentially leading to death. Epileptic patients may also suffer from stigma, and as a result educational and vocational impairments, which heavily affect their quality of life.[16] Therefore, in addition to an appropriate management and medication approach, a holistic approach must be adopted—one that addresses social, educational, and psychological issues that the patient may face.

Later in this book, we also look into "Myasthenia gravis" (MG) as an autoimmune disorder of the neuromuscular junction, which is hallmarked by fatigability and weakness of all striated muscles. A health care provider is likely to encounter more than one patient with this disease throughout their career, as approximately 1 in 10,000 people carry the condition.[17] The manifestation of MG influences practitioners' approach toward treatment of patients requiring special management considerations in order to ensure safe and optimal treatment. MG is an autoimmune neuromuscular disorder marked by fluctuating degrees of weakness of the voluntary (skeletal) muscles of the body, with deterioration during periods of action and improvement following periods of rest.[18]

In the final chapter, we describe and discuss a commonly occurring medical and dental condition, "Facial Palsy." The facial nerve (cranial nerve VII) is composed of two roots, a motor and sensory root.[19] The large motor root carries the motor fibers to the muscles of facial expression and mastication. The sensory root carries general sensory fibers to parts of the external ear and the special sensation of taste. Facial paralysis varies depending on the level of facial nerve lesion. This phenomenon can be reversed spontaneously or via clinical or surgical treatment. About 20% of patients develop some form of sequelae, with unilateral and bilateral complete paralysis of facial muscle movements being the most severe outcome.[20] The global annual incidence of facial paralysis is approximately 70 cases per 100,000. Management for facial paralysis can vary broadly. This is due to the complex etiological nature of the condition. The most common cause for facial paralysis, Bell palsy, is an idiopathic disease that can only be diagnosed by exclusion, and the treatment plans depend on cause and severity of injury.[21]

Overall, there are currently no curative treatments available; however, several therapeutic drugs are being tested in clinical trials.

Current treatment options for these neurological and neurodegenerative diseases, such as disease-modifying drugs or symptomatic therapies, help to manage symptoms and slow the progression of some of the diseases or relieve specific symptoms.

Therefore, multidisciplinary clinical coordination is essential for optimizing health care delivery, increasing survival rate, and enhancing the quality of life of these patients. Modifications to dental treatment are required to ensure the comfort and protection of patients. Home care oral hygiene and regular dentist visits, for example, should occur more frequently due to a higher risk of developing oral diseases.

From a large list of neurological diseases, in this book we aim to describe and discuss Parkinson disease (PD), multiple sclerosis (MS), amyotrophic lateral sclerosis (ALS), Alzheimer disease (AD), cerebrovascular accident (CVA) or stroke, epilepsy (and other seizure disorders), myasthenia gravis (MG), and facial paralysis, which are more commonly seen. We hope that this book offers medical and dental practitioners the required general understanding of the background and description of these neurological diseases, their epidemiology, pathogenesis and etiology, and their potential genetic components. Later, we also describe how the identification, medical history, physical examination, and laboratory testing of these diseases can help in the process of their medical management and treatment approaches. Then we focus on special management of the patients in a dental care setting, prior to and during dental treatment, while considering oral medicine aspects of those conditions. Coordination between physicians, dentists, and other health care providers is suggested and described in the final part of each chapter.

References

[1] Kalia LV, Lang AE. Parkinson's disease. Lancet 2015;386 (9996):896–912

[2] Lees AJ, Hardy J, Revesz T. Parkinson's disease. Lancet. 2009; 373(9680):2055–2066

[3] Yarnall A, Archibald N, Burn D. Parkinson's disease. Medicine (Baltimore). 2012; 40(10):529–535

[4] Compston A, Coles A. Multiple sclerosis. Lancet. 2008; 372 (9648):1502–1517

[5] Hemmer B, Cepok S, Nessler S, Sommer N. Pathogenesis of multiple sclerosis: an update on immunology. Curr Opin Neurol. 2002; 15(3):227–231

[6] Hellings N, Raus J, Stinissen P. Insights into the immunopathogenesis of multiple sclerosis. Immunol Res. 2002; 25(1):27–51

[7] Rolak LA. Multiple sclerosis: it's not the disease you thought it was. Clin Med Res. 2003; 1(1):57–60

[8] Vaughn CB, Jakimovski D, Kavak KS, et al. Epidemiology and treatment of multiple sclerosis in elderly populations. Nat Rev Neurol. 2019; 15(6):329–342

[9] Al-Chalabi A, Hardiman O. The epidemiology of ALS: a conspiracy of genes, environment and time. Nat Rev Neurol. 2013; 9(11):617–628

[10] Brites D, Vaz AR. Microglia centered pathogenesis in ALS: insights in cell interconnectivity. Front Cell Neurosci. 2014; 8:117

[11] Winter Y, Korchounov A, Zhukova TV, Bertschi NE. Depression in elderly patients with Alzheimer dementia or vascular dementia and its influence on their quality of life. J Neurosci Rural Pract. 2011; 2(1):27–32

[12] Qiu C, Kivipelto M, von Strauss E. Epidemiology of Alzheimer's disease: occurrence, determinants, and strategies toward intervention. Dialogues Clin Neurosci. 2009; 11(2):111–128

[13] Hankey GJ. Stroke. Lancet. 2017; 389(10069):641–654

[14] Cooke M, Cuddy MA, Farr B, Moore PA. Cerebrovascular accident under anesthesia during dental surgery. Anesth Prog. 2014; 61(2):73–77

[15] Appleton R, Nicolson A, Chadwick D, MacKenzie J, Smith D. Atlas of Epilepsy. CRC Press; 2006

[16] Knake S, Hamer HM, Rosenow F. Status epilepticus: a critical review. Epilepsy Behav. 2009; 15(1):10–14

[17] McCullough M. Treatment of myasthenia gravis. Australian Prescriber 2007;30(6):160

[18] Yarom N, Barnea E, Nissan J, Gorsky M. Dental management of patients with myasthenia gravis: a literature review. Oral Surg Oral Med Oral Pathol Oral Radiol Endod. 2005; 100(2):158–163

[19] Baker Eric SM. Head and Neck Anatomy for Dental Medicine. Thieme; 2010

[20] Batista KT. Paralisia facial: análise epidemiológica em hospital de reabilitação. Rev Bras Cir Plást. 2011; 26:591–595

[21] Das AK, Sabarigirish K, Kashyap RC. Facial nerve paralysis: a three year retrospective study. Indian J Otolaryngol Head Neck Surg. 2006; 58(3):225–228

2 Parkinson Disease

Armin Ariana

Abstract

Parkinson disease is a chronic neuropathological disorder involving progressive degeneration of dopaminergic and non-dopaminergic neurons in the substantia nigra. It is a prevalent neurological condition affecting 2 to 3% of the population aged 65 years and older. Loss of voluntary motor control, bradykinesia, resting tremor, muscular rigidity, and postural instability are a few symptoms that are particularly experienced by the patients. These motor symptoms are collectively termed "parkinsonism" and are used as cardinal signs for diagnosis by clinicians. Due to the physical limitations in these patients and the systemic manifestations of the disease, health practitioners can play a critical role in assisting them with the maintenance of their oral health and overall well-being. Implementation of an appropriate communicating medium for coordination between dentists and physicians can help in the delivery of an optimal treatment that they provide.

Keywords: Parkinson disease, PD, epidemiology, pathogenesis, oral manifestations, medical management, treatment

2.1 Background of Parkinson Disease

Parkinson disease (PD) is a prevalent neurological condition that affects 2 to 3% of the population aged 65 years and older.[1] Patients with PD are particularly prone to oral diseases due to the physical limitations imposed on them, as well as the systemic manifestations of the disease that interfere with normal salivary functions.[2,3] Dentists, therefore, play a critical role in assisting these patients with maintenance of their oral health and overall well-being. As the population ages, dentists will inevitably encounter more patients with PD, and in order to provide proper dental care and suitable preventative measures, it is of extreme importance that dentists have a thorough understanding of the epidemiology, pathogenesis, oral manifestations, medical management, and treatment of PD.[4]

2.2 Description of Parkinson Disease

Parkinson disease is a chronic neuropathological disorder involving progressive degeneration of dopaminergic and non-dopaminergic neurons present in the substantia nigra.[5] This neuronal degenerative activity causes a loss of voluntary motor control, and patients develop characteristic motor symptoms—bradykinesia, resting tremor, muscular rigidity, and postural instability—which were first described as "shaking palsy" in 1817 by James Parkinson, after whom the disease is named.[5,6] These motor symptoms are collectively termed "parkinsonism" nowadays and are used as cardinal signs for diagnosis by clinicians.[7]

Although commonly classified as a motor disorder, the manifestation of Parkinson disease is, in fact, multisystemic and a range of nonmotor symptoms are also presented by patients. These include cognitive impairment, insomnia, dementia, psychiatric disturbances, and autonomic failures.[8,9] These multisystemic manifestations drastically diminish the patient's quality of life as they induce many detrimental secondary complications, including gastrointestinal, cardiovascular, urinary, and thermoregulatory dysfunctions that arise from dysautonomia.[10,11,12] Various psychiatric disorders that manifest due to the lack of the neurotransmitter, dopamine, are prevalent nonmotor symptoms experienced by many parkinsonian patients, and they encompass depression, psychosis, and loss of impulse control.[13,14,15] The association of these psychiatric conditions with poorer outcomes of the disease has also been found.[13]

As the degenerative progression manifests throughout the course of the disease, patients develop more severe symptoms, and as a consequence, many aspects of the patients' health are compromised. Unfortunately, in spite of the advance of contemporary medical technology, Parkinson disease is, still, an incurable condition, and none of the treatments available can slow down the degenerative process.[7]

2.3 Epidemiology of Parkinson Disease

Parkinson disease affects approximately 0.1 to 0.3% of the world's population.[16,17] One percent of the population older than 60 years are diagnosed with PD.[17,18] Results from epidemiological studies estimate the mean age among PD patients to be 70.6 years,[18] and PD is rarely present in individuals below the age of 50.[8,16,18] Where onset does occur before 50, the disease is classified as early onset Parkinson disease. This is rare, and it occurs in approximately 4% of cases.[16]

The prevalence of Parkinson disease is rising exponentially with age across the globe.[17] By virtue of the growing aging population that benefit from improved quality of life and medical advances, it is expected that the number of PD cases will continue to increase. The life expectancy of the population has increased with the advances in medical facilities, and therefore, it is expected that the number of PD cases will continue to increase. About 10 to 50 per 100,000 people in a given population are being newly diagnosed with Parkinson disease each year, and it is predicted that numbers will double by 2030.[16] Given that this disease occurs primarily in the older population, it is more common in developed countries as a result of longer average life expectancy.[8]

Age by no means is the only contributing factor to this disease. A key role of epidemiology is to translate data and statistics into the knowledge of common risk factors, progression, and prognosis in populations. Epidemiological studies have identified genetic, environmental, and lifestyle factors as likely causes of PD progression,[8] while little to no

significant relationship has been established with gender. Research shows approximately 10 to 15% of patients have a family history of PD,[19] caused by monogenic mutations inherited through autosomal dominant and recessive patterns.[20] The remaining majority of those clinically diagnosed are sporadic cases, likely due to a combination of environmental and genetic factors, with no family history.[7]

Gender roles do not substantially affect the susceptibility of acquiring PD. Some studies report higher prevalence in men than women with a ratio of 1.5:1,[21,22] while other studies lack to show significant differences.[17] Parkinson disease affects all races and nationalities indiscriminately. Studies have yet to find a direct link between nationalities and prevalence of Parkinson disease. For example, Africa had reported a lower prevalence of PD cases than America yet African American and Caucasians in the United States are equally likely to develop this disease.[16,23,24] While not as significant in its contribution to the disease, the prevalence of PD varies between cultures and ethnic groups. In particular, certain genetic mutations are more prevalent in certain ethnic groups. It is thought this may be due to varying environmental factors, and distribution of susceptible genes within the gene pool of the population.[17] It appears that behavioral, genetic, and environmental factors play a larger role in the development of disease rather than gender and race.

The deleterious effect of PD in which clinical symptoms worsen with age was clearly seen when a follow-up of PD patients in a study showed a mean survival rate of 12.6 years after onset.[16] Due to the latent nature of Parkinson disease at onset, accurate diagnosis can pose a challenge. Variations and discrepancies of data collected in epidemiological studies can be ascribed to the difficulty in detection and diagnosis of PD, different methods of data collection, and necessary meticulous follow-up processes with patients and families.[25] Nevertheless, studies on the prevalence, progress, and patterns of PD in population groups lead to better knowledge of this disease in hopes to find a cure in the future.

2.4 Etiology and Pathogenesis of Parkinson Disease

2.4.1 Etiology of Parkinson Disease

Although the etiology of Parkinson disease (PD) is unknown, it is believed to be multifactorial and is likely to involve a complex interaction of environmental and genetic factors (▶ Fig. 2.1).

Traditionally, environmental factors, especially exposure to pesticides and herbicides, have demonstrated a strong association with the onset of PD, due to its dopaminergic neuron toxicity.[26] Rural residency, farming, and consumption of well water appears to increase the risk of PD and may provide further evidence in support of herbicides or pesticide as critical etiological factors.[26]

Several other environmental factors may also be considered as risk contributors of PD. Specifically, a history of head injury has been observed with PD in later life. Non-smokers and non-caffeinated beverage drinkers are believed at higher risk. Further, low blood uric acid levels tend to be associated with increased risk of PD. The mechanisms by which these contribute to PD remain unknown.[27]

Recent research has been focused on the genetic factors involved. Around 15% of individuals with PD have a first-degree relative

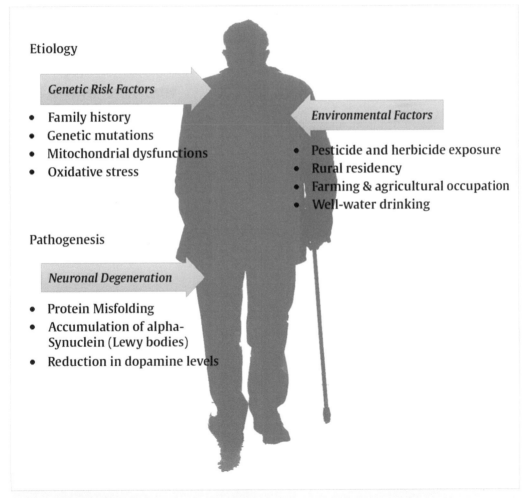

Etiology

Genetic Risk Factors

- Family history
- Genetic mutations
- Mitochondrial dysfunctions
- Oxidative stress

Environmental Factors

- Pesticide and herbicide exposure
- Rural residency
- Farming & agricultural occupation
- Well-water drinking

Pathogenesis

Neuronal Degeneration

- Protein Misfolding
- Accumulation of alpha-Synuclein (Lewy bodies)
- Reduction in dopamine levels

Fig. 2.1 Etiology and pathogenesis of Parkinson disease.

also suffering from the same condition.[27] Several studies of familial PD show inheritance patterns of both autosomal dominant and recessive.[26,27] Several twin studies suggest an increased concordance rate of early onset PD in monozygotic twins.[26,27,28]

Genetic mutations implicated in the development of PD are often involved in protein handling, oxidative stress, and mitochondrial function, including *LRRK2, SNCA, PINK1, PARK7, GBA, DJ1, PARK2*.[29] Again, one or several mutations in these genes alone does not determine the onset. A combination of these genetic mutations with environmental factors could affect age of onset, severity, and progression in a way that has yet to be defined.

2.4.2 Pathogenesis of Parkinson Disease

The typical characteristics of PD are neuronal cell death in the basal ganglia and formation of Lewy bodies in the damaged cells. Lewy bodies are insoluble protein inclusions that are formed through the abnormal accumulation of α-synuclein bound to ubiquitin.[26] The *SNCA* gene mentioned earlier as a genetic etiological factor encodes α-synuclein, and therefore mutation of this gene increases the risk of PD. Lewy bodies start accumulating in the substantia nigra, which is in the region of the midbrain, then spread to the basal forebrain and finally occupy the neocortex, signifying the main sites of neuron degeneration in PD.[26] The loss of neurons also causes a great reduction in dopamine levels in the regions mentioned above. The brain uses dopamine as neurotransmitters, and reduction poses inhibition of the dopamine pathway, affecting reward-motivated behaviors and motor control.[26,30]

Mitochondrial dysfunction and oxidative stress are closely interlinked in the pathogenesis of PD. Their importance has been reinforced by identification of gene mutations that induce dopaminergic cell death in some familial and sporadic PD cases.[27] Mitochondrial dysfunction involves deficiencies of respiratory chain proteins, most commonly respiratory chain protein complex I. This dysfunction can result from etiological genetic factors that encode mitochondrial proteins, for example, *PINK1, DJ1*, and *parkin*.[26] *PINK1* encodes PTEN-induced putative kinase I that protects neuronal cells from stress-related mitochondrial dysfunction.[26] It induces autophagy of depolarized mitochondria through the binding of parkin protein.[26] As a result of this, mutations in this gene contribute to autosomal recessive PD. Patients with *PINK1* mutation show nigrostriatal neuron cell loss and Lewy body formation. Environmental agents can also influence its function. The relationship between mitochondrial dysfunction and oxidative stress can be seen as reciprocal. Dopaminergic neurons are especially sensitive to calcium ion imbalance. Accumulation of intracellular calcium through voltage-dependent channels would result in an increase of mitochondrial free radicals and contribute to neuron death.[27,29]

Another common abnormality of PD can be manifested as proteasome inhibition. Alteration in the expression of subunits and regulatory cap induces a different organization of proteasomes, thus reducing proteasomal enzyme activity, and eventually, loss of nigral dopaminergic neurons. This degradation is achieved by a cascade of ATP-dependent peptidases.[30] Proteasome degradation has shown a strong association with mitochondrial dysfunction and oxidative stress. Free radicals impair mitochondrial respiratory chain function and increase substrate load on proteasomes.[29] Abnormal proteins then accumulate in the cytosol due to proteasome degradation. This poses potential acceleration in neuron cell dysfunction and death.

2.5 Genetic Component of Parkinson Disease

Parkinson disease is a multifactorial neurodegenerative disorder. It can be either familial or sporadic.[7] In the majority of cases, Parkinson disease occurs due to sporadic causes resulting from the interplay of both genetic mutations and environmental exposures.[7] While the nature of the genetic involvement in PD requires further research, it is well recognized as having considerable involvement in the onset, progression, and clinical symptoms of the disease.[1,31] Whether familial or sporadic, the same pattern of dopaminergic neuron degeneration in the substantia nigra occurs.[31]

Currently, 26 genetic variations and gene loci have been identified as contributing to the risk of Parkinson disease.[32] Of these, there are six known monogenic forms of PD, accounting for 3 to 5% of sporadic and 30% of familial cases.[1,20] Inheritance follows both autosomal-dominant and autosomal-recessive patterns. The scope of research into these monogenic mutations and their relationship to Parkinson disease is outlined below.

2.5.1 Autosomal-Dominant Mutations

There are currently three genes associated with autosomal-dominant monogenic forms of Parkinson disease: SNCA, LRRK2, and VPS35.[32]

The first gene linked to PD was that of SNCA: a 140-amino acid protein encoding for α-synuclein. As mentioned above, mutations in this gene include point, duplications, and triplications, and follow an autosomal-dominant pattern of inheritance. Mutated SNCA produces a form of α-synuclein that is misfolded, insoluble, and contributes to PD pathogenesis by aggregating in the cell bodies and processes of neurons as inclusions, forming a substantial component of Lewy bodies and neurites, respectively.[7] On its own, α-synuclein does not produce such effects but is toxic in these excess aggregations.[7,33]

A hallmark characteristic in the progression of Parkinson disease is an accumulation of aggregated α-synuclein and the resulting Lewy body pathology. This follows specific patterns as the disease progresses.[34] The SNCA mutation itself causes an early onset, rapidly progressing form of Parkinson disease, which has been associated with both familial and sporadic cases.[1]

The most common genetic mutation in Parkinson disease occurs in leucine-rich repeat kinase 2 (LRRK2), which accounts for 1% of sporadic and 4% of familial occurrences.[7] This mutation results in a form of the disease with the mid-late onset and slow progression.[7] The LRRK2 protein is involved in "neurite outgrowth, synaptic morphogenesis, membrane trafficking, autophagy and protein synthesis."[7] Eight mutations of LRRK2 have been linked to PD, with the Gly2019Ser substitution being the most common.[7] LRRK2-induced Parkinson disease is highly prevalent in North African Arab and Ashkenazi Jew ethnic groups, accounting for 30% of familial, 13% of sporadic and 37% of familial, and 41% of sporadic cases, respectively.[7]

The final monogenic form of PD inherited through autosomal-dominant patterns is VPS35 (vacuolar protein sorting 35 retromolar complex). This protein is responsible for transporting proteins between endosomes and the Golgi apparatus.[32] It causes late-onset PD.

2.5.2 Autosomal-Recessive Mutations

Recessively inherited Parkinson disease has been linked to monogenic mutations in Parkin, PINK1, and DJ-1. It can be the result of homozygous or compound heterozygous mutations.[32] These genes are all associated with mitochondrial health and quality control, which provides further support for mitochondrial dysfunction as a cause of the disease.[20,35] Recessively inherited Parkinson disease is always associated with early onset.

Parkin, encoding for E3 ubiquitin ligase, was the second gene linked to PD, and the first to be associated with recessive inheritance.[20] It is the most common genetic cause of recessively inherited PD.[20] In early onset patients, it accounts for 50% of familial and 15% of sporadic cases.[7,36] The resulting clinical phenotype is associated with early onset and slow progression.

PINK1 encodes for phosphatase and tensin homolog-induced putative kinase 1. This mutation accounts for 1 to 8% of sporadic PD cases. It is involved in mitochondrial calcium homeostasis and results in Parkinson disease with early onset and slow progression.[20,35]

DJ-1 (Parkinson disease protein 7) accounts for 1 to 2% of early onset cases. The protein produced is involved in protecting against oxidative stress.[20,35]

Genetic involvement in Parkinson disease is well founded and known to have a substantial role in the development of the disease. Further research into the nature of the genetic involvement of Parkinson disease will provide greater insight into the characteristics, pathogenesis, and progression of individual cases, improve patient prognosis, and assist in the development of more targeted treatment options.

2.6 Diagnostic Evaluation of Parkinson Disease

2.6.1 Clinical Features of Parkinson Disease

Parkinson disease is characterized by a wide range of motor and nonmotor symptoms that affect and impair function to variable degrees —depending on the onset and severity of disease, which advances with time (▶ Fig. 2.2).

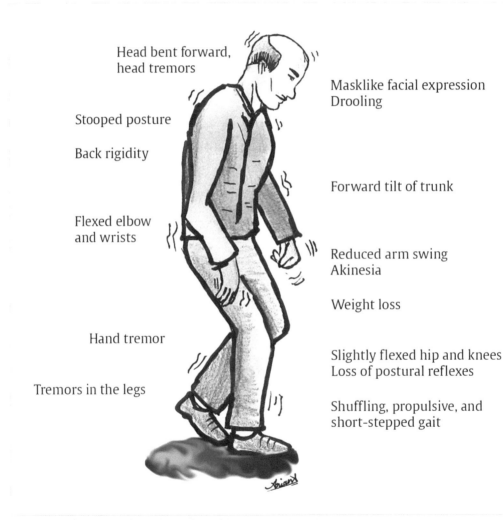

Head bent forward, head tremors

Stooped posture

Back rigidity

Flexed elbow and wrists

Hand tremor

Tremors in the legs

Masklike facial expression
Drooling

Forward tilt of trunk

Reduced arm swing
Akinesia

Weight loss

Slightly flexed hip and knees
Loss of postural reflexes

Shuffling, propulsive, and short-stepped gait

Fig. 2.2 Parkinson disease presentation.

There are four classic symptoms of Parkinson disease: muscular rigidity, bradykinesia, tremor at rest, and postural instability. Other significant parkinsonian symptoms include postural deformities and gait disturbance, such as freezing.[37]

Bradykinesia

Bradykinesia is defined as the slowness of movement and has been identified as the most characteristic manifestation of Parkinson disease.[37] It is a distinctive feature of basal ganglia disorders and may also be observed in other conditions. Those affected will display slow movement in performing daily activities and diminished reaction times. They may also experience difficulties with planning and executing movements, multitasking, or performing tasks that involve fine motor control. Other features of bradykinesia include loss of facial expression, decreased reflex, and spontaneous movements and drooling as a result of impaired swallowing.[37] Assessment involves rapid and sequential tapping of fingers, and rapid heel taps—slowness and reduced amplitude indicate bradykinesia.[38]

Muscular Rigidity

Rigidity is observed with increased resistance when flexing, extending, or rotating about a joint.[37] Physicians often test for this within the patient's cubital fossa or with wrist supination or pronation.[38] Resistance can be identified as lead-pipe rigidity, characterized by increased tone and hence continuous rigidity, or cogwheel rigidity, which occurs with underlying tremor and is characterized by a catch-and-release effect.[38] Pain may also be presented with rigidity, which can occur proximally and distally.[37]

Resting Tremor

This is the most common and easily identified feature of Parkinson disease.[37] It is important that resting tremor is distinguished from postural or kinetic tremor, which may be more indicative of essential tremor.[38] Resting tremors in Parkinson disease are unilateral and occur at a frequency of 4 to 6 Hz.[37] It is commonly observed when patients' hands are resting in their lap and demonstrate pill-rolling (supination-pronation) tremors.[38] Resting tremor can also be observed in the chin, jaw, lips, and legs; however, it rarely presents in the neck, head, or voice, which more often indicates essential tremor.[37]

Postural Instability

Postural instability usually manifests in later stages of Parkinson disease as it results from the loss of postural reflexes and the onset of earlier clinical symptoms.[37] It is assessed using the pull test to evaluate the patient's postural response by observing the degree of retropulsion or propulsion when the patient is pulled backward or forward rapidly by the shoulders. An abnormal postural response is identified when the patient takes more than two steps backwards or with the absence of any postural response.[37] Together with gait disturbances, postural instability is a significant cause of loss of balance and falls.[38]

Nonmotor Features

In addition to the identification of motor symptoms for clinical diagnosis of Parkinson disease, there is now increased attention and emphasis on the importance of nonmotor symptoms, although often poorly recognized (▶ Fig. 2.3).[39] Despite the focus on identification of motor symptoms, studies have shown the greater importance of nonmotor symptoms when assessing quality of life, health economics, or institutionalization rates.[39] Nonmotor symptoms involve cognitive and neurobehavioral abnormalities, autonomic dysfunction, sleep disorders, and sensory abnormalities. Some of the common symptoms include depression, constipation, cognitive impairment, sexual dysfunction, rapid eye movement, sleep behavior disorder, and olfactory problems.[37] Although nonmotor symptoms may present in the earlier stages of disease, studies have found manifestation generally increases with advancing age and

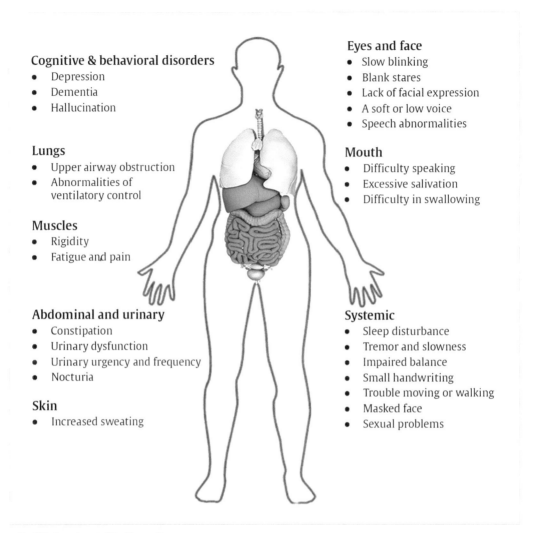

Cognitive & behavioral disorders
- Depression
- Dementia
- Hallucination

Lungs
- Upper airway obstruction
- Abnormalities of ventilatory control

Muscles
- Rigidity
- Fatigue and pain

Abdominal and urinary
- Constipation
- Urinary dysfunction
- Urinary urgency and frequency
- Nocturia

Skin
- Increased sweating

Eyes and face
- Slow blinking
- Blank stares
- Lack of facial expression
- A soft or low voice
- Speech abnormalities

Mouth
- Difficulty speaking
- Excessive salivation
- Difficulty in swallowing

Systemic
- Sleep disturbance
- Tremor and slowness
- Impaired balance
- Small handwriting
- Trouble moving or walking
- Masked face
- Sexual problems

Fig. 2.3 Symptoms of Parkinson disease.

severity of disease. Therefore, the identification and treatment of nonmotor symptoms become increasingly important with increased average age and life expectancy.[39]

2.6.2 Diagnosis of Parkinson Disease

Correct diagnosis of disease is essential for increased precision in prognosis, effective treatment, and clinical research. However, there is currently no definitive clinical diagnostic test, such as laboratory tests or imaging studies, that confirms diagnosis for Parkinson disease.[37] Clinical diagnosis remains through the identification of clinical symptoms, physical examination, and careful history taking, along with the use of clinical criteria.[40] The UK Parkinson Disease Brain Bank criteria used in clinic and clinical research has shown improvements in accuracy of diagnosis—with diagnostic specificity and sensitivity estimated at 98.6 and 91.1%, respectively.[40] However, up to 10% of diagnoses will have to be reevaluated at post-mortem examinations.[40] Neuropathological assessment on autopsy has been considered the gold standard for diagnosis of Parkinson disease[37]—identification of neuronal loss in the substantia nigra pars compacta (SNpc), the presence of Lewy bodies in surviving SNpc neurons, and no other pathological evidence indicative of other parkinsonian diseases.[7]

2.6.3 Clinical Differential Diagnosis of Parkinson Disease

Diagnosis of Parkinson disease may be considered a straightforward clinical assessment of patients who present with typical symptoms of parkinsonism and demonstrate improvement with levodopa treatment.[40] However, with overlapping signs and symptoms, differentiating Parkinson disease from other forms of Parkinsonism may be difficult and cause misdiagnosis.[37] This may be particularly challenging in the earlier stages of disease with greater overlap of symptoms.[40] However, with increasing knowledge of the various forms of Parkinsonism, diagnostic accuracy has greatly improved. Common causes for misdiagnosis include the presence of essential tremor, drug-induced tremor, atypical parkinsonian syndromes, vascular parkinsonism, Alzheimer disease, and dementia with Lewy bodies.[40]

Essential Tremor

Essential tremor may cause symptoms of bilateral and symmetrical postural or kinetic tremor. Tremors can be observed and appear persistent while affecting the hands and forearms. Symptoms of postural tremor in essential tremor are visible immediately when arms are outstretched without latency, whereas postural tremor in Parkinson disease is more characteristic of re-emergent tremor, which is only apparent after some latency after outstretching the arms. Some additional differentiating features include sensitivity to alcohol, which is indicative of essential tremor, and sensitivity to levodopa, which is more characteristic of Parkinson disease.[40]

Vascular Parkinsonism

Vascular parkinsonism occurs in patients with cerebrovascular disease and is characteristic of widespread bilateral lacunar infarcts. Onset occurs gradually and causes parkinsonian gait disorder that presents with symptoms of small stepped gait and freezing.[40]

Drug-induced Parkinsonism

Drug-induced parkinsonism can be caused by long-term use of various anti-dopaminergic drugs, in which antipsychotics and antiemetics are the most common causes. Clinicians may experience difficulty in differential diagnosis as drug-induced parkinsonism can cause symptoms that present identical to features of Parkinson disease. Some symptoms favoring the diagnosis of drug-induced parkinsonism are the presence of orofacial dyskinesia or akathisia. Diagnosis may be particularly challenging in patients with unclear drug history or with patients taking only small quantities of medication. Patients who do not show regression of parkinsonism after withdrawal of drugs may be indicative of underlying Parkinson disease.[40]

2.7 Medical Management and Treatment of Parkinson Disease

2.7.1 Common Drugs Used

Since Parkinson disease is closely linked to a depletion of dopamine in the CNS[41] and an imbalance of acetylcholine and dopamine in the basal ganglia, increasing the level of dopamine is considered as the essential drug treatment of Parkinson disease. A major obstacle here is that dopamine cannot cross the blood–brain barrier (BBB). For this reason, Levodopa is used as the gold standard drug.[41] As the precursor to dopamine, Levodopa travels from the gastrointestinal system into peripheral tissues, and a small amount of Levodopa (less than 1%) crosses the BBB into the CNS and is converted into dopamine by decarboxylation.[42] In the CNS, dopamine acts on D1 dopamine receptors, which are the most abundant, as well as the D2 receptors, which are located presynaptically.[43] In peripheral tissues, Levodopa is converted into dopamine by dopa decarboxylase. This will lead to side effects such as postural nausea, postural hypotension, anxiety, and cardiac arrhythmias. In clinical practice, Levodopa is always used with Carbidopa or Benserazide (peripheral decarboxylase inhibitors) to minimize peripheral side effects and decrease the dose of Levodopa.[42]

Central anticholinergics such as Benztropine, Benzhexol, and Biperiden are less effective than Levodopa.[41] They act by inhibiting acetylcholine and are used as an adjunctive therapy to control drug-induced extrapyramidal disorders.[41] Amantadine, as a dopamine facilitator, enhances the release of dopamine and inhibits reuptake of dopamine. While less effective than Levodopa, it is more effective than anticholinergics.[41] Dopaminergic agonists are also used to treat Parkinson disease. Bromocriptine is used in the later stages of Parkinson disease as a potent D_2 agonist, while Ropinirole and Pramipexole are supplementary drugs to Levodopa in advanced cases. These drugs have a longer duration than Levodopa and often are used to manage dose-related fluctuations.[42]

2.7.2 Adverse Effects of Drugs and Drug Management

The adverse effects of Levodopa include choreiform movements, dystonic movements, nausea, vomiting, postural hypotension, cardiac arrhythmias, alteration of taste sensation, mild anxiety, nightmares, and mental confusion.[41] An "On-Off" phenomenon usually occurs after taking Levodopa for two or more years. Here, the patient alternates between states of improved clinical conditions and the loss of therapeutic effects.[41] The management of this issue could be improved by taking a "drug holiday," whereby the patient stops taking Levodopa treatment for 4 to 15 days, then gradually increases the dose.[41]

2.7.3 Drug Delivery Method

Although oral administration is more commonly used for Levodopa and other drugs, there are also some advantages to nonoral routes of drug administration. For instance, subcutaneous and transdermal routes of administration can ensure a constant, rate-controlled drug delivery and reduce drug toxicity and fluctuations.[44] Continuous subcutaneous infusion of apomorphine produces improvement of severe motor complications.[44] However, long-term apomorphine infusion can lead to cutaneous reactions such as bruises, rashes, or nodules.[44]

2.7.4 Other Therapies and Social Support

In general, surgery is recommended when drug treatment fails. Deep brain stimulation benefits patients with early onset Parkinson disease and patients who have experienced long-term on-off effects of the disease.[45] Other surgery options include lesional surgery, which is an alternative to deep brain stimulation; pallidotomy, which is appropriate for severe dyskinesia; and thalamic deep brain surgery, mainly for controlling tremors.[45]

To provide optimal care to patients, a carer support network is required. Parkinson disease nurse specialists, physiotherapists, speech therapists, and occupational therapists can work collaboratively with the patients to achieve a good result. A healthy diet is also suggested, such as eating plenty of fruits and vegetables in the early stages of the disease.

2.8 Management of Dental Patients with Parkinson Disease

Many special considerations need to be taken in order to manage the symptoms of PD patients during dental treatment. The first treatment consideration for a PD patient undergoing dental treatment is to schedule the appointment early in the morning and 60 to 90 minutes after the patient has taken their medication. This will allow for treatment when medication is at its most effective and when the patient is least affected by their symptoms.[46] The patient should also empty their bladder before the appointment, as PD may adversely affect urinary retention,[47] and attend the appointment with a caregiver whenever possible.

Once the patient has entered the dental clinic, the operator should be mindful of the possibility of neurogenic orthostatic hypotension[48] and assist them in slowly moving into and out of the dental chair. In addition, to lessen any difficulties with swallowing, the dental chair should not be inclined too far backward.[49] The constant use of a high-speed suction or saliva ejector may also minimize any incidences of drooling, and the placement of a rubber dam will minimize the higher risk of aspiration in PD patients.[50] Tremors and muscle rigidity may cause poor lip closure, uncontrolled movements of the jaw, and difficulties with keeping the mouth open, so intraoral bite blocks, mouth props, and head stabilization may be useful to facilitate safe access to the mouth.[49]

During the appointment, the patient may have difficulty with verbal and nonverbal communication, so the operator should communicate with the patient through gentle responses and closed questions in order to improve the flow of information during the appointment.[51] Complications such as an increased caries and periodontal disease risk, increased probability of fractured and attrited teeth, and increased risk of temporomandibular joint disorders should be discussed with the patient, and the operator should observe for such issues in the patient.[48] Subsequently, the patient should receive advice about ways in which they can minimize the impact of their bradykinesia, tremors, and muscle rigidity on their oral health. Supplementary tools that minimize the dependence on manual dexterity to perform personal oral care, such as electric toothbrushes, special toothbrushes, interdental brushes, and fluoride mouthwashes, can be recommended for use by the patient.[51]

In order to address concerns related to xerostomia or an increased risk of dental caries, topical application of a high concentration fluoride product to the teeth may be performed during the appointment, especially if there is evidence of early demineralization of the tooth enamel.[49] Patients suffering from xerostomia should be advised to sip water throughout the day; chew sugar-free gum containing xylitol to stimulate salivary flow; use saliva substitutes; avoid candies containing sucrose; and use fluoridated mouthwash.[52] If there are issues with dentition or periodontal structures in the early stages of PD, it is best to treat them before the disease progresses and the patient experiences further degeneration of motor function.[47] Lastly, in order to strengthen the support received by the patient with regard to their daily maintenance of teeth and gum tissue, caregivers should be educated about the importance of their involvement in the maintenance of the patient's oral health. The operator is encouraged to provide instructions regarding proper oral hygiene management to both the patient and caregiver, and to also demonstrate to the caregiver the placement of topical sodium fluoride products to the patient's teeth.[50]

2.9 Oral Medicine Aspects of Parkinson Disease

2.9.1 Orofacial Complications of Parkinson Disease

Parkinson disease is associated with a lack of facial expression, which is sometimes referred to as "mask-like" face. This symptom results from the reduction in movements of small facial muscles, reduction in blinking rate, trembling of the forehead, eyelids, tongue and lips, and involuntary movement of the mandible. Normally, patients with Parkinson disease have eyesight weakness and difficulties in reading.[53] Hyposmia or anosmia is reported in some patients with Parkinson disease, which is probably because of loss of neurons in the anterior olfactory nucleus.[54]

The loss of proper motor control of the tongue and pharynx disrupts the wavelike contraction of the smooth muscle of digestive tract, leading to difficulty in swallowing and inability to form a bolus. In addition to this, the discomfort of the tongue, the floor of the mouth, lips, and cheeks, as well as difficulty in closing the mouth are experienced by PD patients.[55,56] These symptoms present in approximately 75% of patients suffering from

PD and, with the improper forward positioning of the head, subsequently cause drooling of saliva from the corners of the mouth—this is often associated with angular cheilosis, skin irritation, and halitosis.[57]

Other oral manifestations of Parkinson disease may include the discomfort of the temporomandibular joint, cracked teeth, attrition, lack of salivary control, soft tissue trauma, difficulty in retaining dentures, and hypophonia (softening of the voice of patient).[54,56] When the disease reaches its later stages, the patient's voice is hardly audible, which is caused by hypokinesia (reduced frequency and amplitude of the movement) of vocal organs.[54]

2.9.2 Parkinson Disease Medications and Adverse Orofacial Effects

Xerostomia and burning mouth are reported among 55 and 24% of PD patients, respectively. Xerostomia is a result of parasympatholytic or antimuscarinic effects of prescribed Parkinson medications. On the other hand, burning mouth can be caused by lack of vitamins and minerals, hormonal imbalances, candida infections, or parafunctional activity. Chronic xerostomia may also cause burning mouth syndrome. High rates of dental caries and exacerbated periodontal disease can be observed when the buffering capacity of saliva reduces. As a result, the sensitivity of taste buds is adversely affected, which may lead to dysgeusia.[56] Nutritional deficiency is another side effect of xerostomia due to esophageal injury.[56] Xerostomia is a known adverse effect of the following PD medications: Amantadine, Benztropine, Cabergoline, Levodopa with Carbidopa, Levodopa with Carbidopa and Entacapone, Rasagiline, Ropinirole, Trihexyphenidyl.[50]

Dysgeusia or parageusia is an abnormality in a patient's ability to detect taste[58] and may be caused by PD medications such as Levodopa with Carbidopa, Levodopa with Carbidopa and Entacapone, and Selegiline.[50]

Gingivitis, or inflammation of the gingiva, is the most common type of periodontal disease, which is caused by the accumulation of plaque on tooth surfaces. Gingivitis is known to be an adverse effect of Ropinirole, one of the medications used to treat PD.[50]

Glossitis is the inflammation of the tongue with loss of papillae, leaving a smooth tongue surface.[59] Glossitis can be caused by Levodopa with Carbidopa, Levodopa with Carbidopa and Entacapone, and Ropinirole.[50]

Tongue edema is swelling of the tongue, normally caused by an allergic reaction or angioedema. The swelling occurs due to fluid accumulation in the tissue of the tongue.[60] Ropinirole can cause tongue edema in Parkinson disease patients.

Bruxism is another adverse effect of PD medications, which Shetty et al define as "a movement disorder characterized by grinding and clenching of teeth."[61] The clinical relevance of this disorder is the potential failure of dental restorations, tooth damage, induction of temporal headache, and temporomandibular disorders.[61] Bruxism is caused by medications such as Levodopa with Carbidopa, Levodopa with Carbidopa and Entacapone, and Selegiline.[50]

Some other miscellaneous adverse side effects of medications used in Parkinson disease treatment can be as follows[50]:
• Toothache: Cabergoline, Ropinirole.
• Burning lips: Selegiline.
• Burning mouth: Selegiline.
• Throat irritation: Cabergoline.
• Periorbital edema: Cabergoline.
• Trismus: Levodopa with Carbidopa, Levodopa with Carbidopa and Entacapone.
• Sialorrhea: Levodopa with Carbidopa, Levodopa with Carbidopa and Entacapone.
• Dark saliva: Levodopa with Carbidopa, Levodopa with Carbidopa and Entacapone.
• Pigmentation of teeth: Levodopa with Carbidopa, Levodopa with Carbidopa and Entacapone.

2.10 Coordination of Care between Dentist and Physician

A vital component in monitoring and treating patients with Parkinson disease is the level of communication and coordination between the dentist, physician, patient, and possibly the caretaker (depending on the severity of the disease). Frequent communication between the dentist and physician allows for greater understanding of the progression of the disease, which in turn allows for a better prognosis and treatment for the patient, such as modifying tooth brushing techniques to accommodate for the deteriorating motor control.[2] Along with knowing the progression of the disease both parties must also coordinate to determine the current stage of the disease, level of cognitive ability, medications, and medication regime as well as any other factors that may need to be taken into account when performing dental treatment. It is also imperative that the dental treatment is performed as early as possible because as PD reaches its later stages, the ability of the patient to cooperate will also decrease, thus creating difficulty in terms of patient compliance.

Parkinson disease harbors a great risk for the development of biofilm due to poor manual dexterity as a result of declining cognitive abilities.[62] This then leads to poorer oral health by inducing the accumulation of plaque, which ultimately leads to dental caries, gingivitis, and periodontitis.[63] Dentists are not only involved in managing the oral health of a patient but must also work in tandem with the physician through a coordinated approach to provide, manage, and maintain the best possible treatment for their patients.[2]

If this coordination of care is neglected, there could be adverse effects on the patient's overall health. A clear example of this would be the effect of certain medication on dental treatment such as the interaction between Warfarin and Ropinirole. If the physician is prescribing a certain medication such as Warfarin (an anticoagulant) and the patient is also receiving Ropinirole, a severe amount of blood loss is expected due to the synergistic blood thinning properties.[64] Thus, restricting the dentist from performing mechanical therapy such as scaling procedures, root canals, and extractions due to the danger of severe blood loss and postural hypotension.[65,66] This indicates the necessity for the dentist to be fully aware of all medications being taken by the patient. Another example of this is displayed through the adverse effects of certain PD medication such as Levodopa which can also cause postural hypotension. This will then require coordination with the patient's physician to reduce the dose of the medication in the short term in order to reduce these adverse effects if they will have a significant impact on the dental treatment being provided.[67]

The carer plays a vital role in the maintenance of the patient's overall health and well-being by relaying critical information about the patient to the dentist and physician once the patient is no longer able to do so by themselves due to their impaired cognitive capability. The legal guardian of the patient has the responsibility to act on behalf of the patient when obtaining consent for certain treatments allowing both parties (physician and dentist) to treat the patient immediately. Granting this permission allows for faster treatment.[2] Therefore, the coordination between the patient, dentist, physician, carer, and legal guardian contains a critical role in maintaining uniformity.

In conclusion, the coordination between dentists and physicians is a significant factor in terms of the treatment in which they can provide. A possible program that could be implemented would be communicating through a medium such as an electronic health portfolio, similar to that which is seen in many medical practices.[68] This would allow both parties to document, adjust, and input information based on the patient's overall health, treatments, and undertaken medications. This way the coordination of care between both parties (dentists and physicians) will be clear, coherent, and updated, which ultimately produces the highest level of care for the patient.

References

[1] Williams-Gray CH, Worth PF. Parkinson's disease. Medicine (Baltimore). 2016; 44(9):542–546
[2] DeBowes SL, Tolle SL, Bruhn AM. Parkinson's disease: considerations for dental hygienists. Int J Dent Hyg. 2013; 11(1): 15–21

[3] Mougeot JL, Hirsch MA, Stevens CB, Mougeot F. Oral biomarkers in exercise-induced neuroplasticity in Parkinson's disease. Oral Dis. 2016; 22(8):745–753

[4] Grover S, Rhodus N. Dental implications of Parkinson disease. Dent Abstr. 2012; 57(6):316–318

[5] Lees AJ, Hardy J, Revesz T. Parkinson's disease. Lancet. 2009; 373(9680):2055–2066

[6] Yarnall A, Archibald N, Burn D. Parkinson's disease. Medicine (Baltimore). 2012; 40(10):529–535

[7] Kalia LV, Lang AE. Parkinson's disease. Lancet. 2015; 386 (9996):896–912

[8] Alves G, Forsaa EB, Pedersen KF, Dreetz Gjerstad M, Larsen JP. Epidemiology of Parkinson's disease. J Neurol. 2008; 255 Suppl 5:18–32

[9] Behari M, Bhattacharyya KB, Borgohain R, et al. Parkinson's disease. Ann Indian Acad Neurol. 2011; 14(5) Suppl 1:S2–S6

[10] Duncan GW, Khoo TK, Yarnall AJ, et al. Health-related quality of life in early Parkinson's disease: the impact of nonmotor symptoms. Mov Disord. 2014; 29(2):195–202

[11] Ziemssen T, Reichmann H. Non-motor dysfunction in Parkinson's disease. Parkinsonism Relat Disord. 2007; 13(6):323–332

[12] Oka H, Toyoda C, Yogo M, Mochio S. Olfactory dysfunction and cardiovascular dysautonomia in Parkinson's disease. J Neurol. 2010; 257(6):969–976

[13] Grover S, Somaiya M, Kumar S, Avasthi A. Psychiatric aspects of Parkinson's disease. J Neurosci Rural Pract. 2015; 6(1):65–76

[14] Weintraub D, Stern MB. Psychiatric complications in Parkinson disease. Am J Geriatr Psychiatry. 2005; 13(10):844–851

[15] Chinta SJ, Andersen JK. Dopaminergic neurons. Int J Biochem Cell Biol. 2005; 37(5):942–946

[16] Elbaz A, Carcaillon L, Kab S, Moisan F. Epidemiology of Parkinson's disease. Rev Neurol (Paris). 2016; 172(1):14–26

[17] de Lau LM, Breteler MM. Epidemiology of Parkinson's disease. Lancet Neurol. 2006; 5(6):525–535

[18] Tysnes OB, Storstein A. Epidemiology of Parkinson's disease. J Neural Transm (Vienna). 2017; 124(8):901–905

[19] Thacker EL, Ascherio A. Familial aggregation of Parkinson's disease: a meta-analysis. Mov Disord. 2008; 23(8):1174–1183

[20] Klein C, Westenberger A. Genetics of Parkinson's disease. Cold Spring Harb Perspect Med. 2012; 2(1):a008888

[21] Taylor KS, Cook JA, Counsell CE. Heterogeneity in male to female risk for Parkinson's disease. J Neurol Neurosurg Psychiatry. 2007; 78(8):905–906

[22] Wooten GF, Currie LJ, Bovbjerg VE, Lee JK, Patrie J. Are men at greater risk for Parkinson's disease than women? J Neurol Neurosurg Psychiatry. 2004; 75(4):637–639

[23] Okubadejo NU, Bower JH, Rocca WA, Maraganore DM. Parkinson's disease in Africa: a systematic review of epidemiologic and genetic studies. Mov Disord. 2006; 21(12):2150–2156

[24] Schoenberg BS, Osuntokun BO, Adeuja AO, et al. Comparison of the prevalence of Parkinson's disease in black populations in the rural United States and in rural Nigeria: door-to-door community studies. Neurology. 1988; 38(4):645–646

[25] Elbaz A, Carcaillon L, Kab S, Moisan F. Epidemiology of Parkinson's disease. Rev Neurol (Paris). 2016; 172(1):14–26

[26] Schapira AH, Jenner P. Etiology and pathogenesis of Parkinson's disease. Mov Disord. 2011; 26(6):1049–1055

[27] Kumar A. Textbook of Movement Disorders. New Delhi, India: Jaypee Brothers Medical Pub Ltd.; 2014

[28] Tanner CM, Ottman R, Goldman SM, et al. Parkinson disease in twins: an etiologic study. JAMA. 1999; 281(4):341–346

[29] Olanow CW, Tatton WG. Etiology and pathogenesis of Parkinson's disease. Annu Rev Neurosci. 1999; 22(1):123–144

[30] Eriksen JL, Wszolek Z, Petrucelli L. Molecular pathogenesis of Parkinson disease. Arch Neurol. 2005; 62(3):353–357

[31] Dickson DW. Parkinson's disease and parkinsonism: neuropathology. Cold Spring Harb Perspect Med. 2012; 2(8): a009258

[32] Lill CM. Genetics of Parkinson's disease. Mol Cell Probes. 2016; 30(6):386–396

[33] Stefanis L. α-Synuclein in Parkinson's disease. Cold Spring Harb Perspect Med. 2012; 2(2):a009399

[34] Trinh J, Farrer M. Advances in the genetics of Parkinson disease. Nat Rev Neurol. 2013; 9(8):445–454

[35] Lubbe S, Morris HR. Recent advances in Parkinson's disease genetics. J Neurol. 2014; 261(2):259–266

[36] Singleton AB, Farrer MJ, Bonifati V. The genetics of Parkinson's disease: progress and therapeutic implications. Mov Disord. 2013; 28(1):14–23

[37] Jankovic J. Parkinson's disease: clinical features and diagnosis. J Neurol Neurosurg Psychiatry. 2008; 79(4):368–376

[38] Rao SS, Hofmann LA, Shakil A. Parkinson's disease: diagnosis and treatment. Am Fam Physician. 2006; 74(12):2046–2054

[39] Chaudhuri KR, Healy DG, Schapira AH, National Institute for Clinical Excellence. Non-motor symptoms of Parkinson's disease: diagnosis and management. Lancet Neurol. 2006; 5(3): 235–245

[40] Tolosa E, Wenning G, Poewe W. The diagnosis of Parkinson's disease. Lancet Neurol. 2006; 5(1):75–86

[41] Acosta WR. Pharmacology for Health Professionals. 2nd ed. Philadelphia, PA: Lippincott Williams & Wilkins; 2013:599

[42] Chabner BA, Knollman B. Goodman & Gilman's The Pharmacological Basis of Therapeutics. 12th ed. The McGraw-Hill Companies; 2011

[43] Rang HP, Ritter JM, Flower RJ, Henderson G. Rang & Dale's Pharmacology. 8th ed. Philadelphia, PA: Elsevier Ltd.; 2016:723

[44] Pfeiffer RF, Wszolek ZK, Ebadi M. Parkinson's Disease. 2nd ed. CRC Press; 2012

[45] Chaudhuri KR, Healy DG, Schapira AH. Fast Facts: Parkinson's Disease. 3rd ed. Health Press Limited; 2011:146

[46] Zlotnik Y, Balash Y, Korczyn AD, Giladi N, Gurevich T. Disorders of the oral cavity in Parkinson's disease and parkinsonian syndromes. Parkinsons Dis. 2015; 2015:379482

[47] Dougall A, Fiske J. Access to special care dentistry, part 9. Special care dentistry services for older people. Br Dent J. 2008; 205(8):421–434

[48] Sánchez-Ferro A, Benito-León J, Gómez-Esteban JC. The management of orthostatic hypotension in Parkinson's disease. Front Neurol. 2013; 4(64):64

[49] Robbins MR, Robbins MR. Neurologic diseases in special care patients. Dent Clin North Am. 2016; 60(3):707–735

[50] Friedlander AH, Mahler M, Norman KM, Ettinger RL. Parkinson disease: systemic and orofacial manifestations, medical and dental management. J Am Dent Assoc. 2009; 140(6): 658–669

[51] Katyayan PA, Katyayan MK, Nugala B. Dental management of Parkinson's disease: a case report. N Y State Dent J. 2013; 79 (5):33–39

[52] Villa A, Connell CL, Abati S. Diagnosis and management of xerostomia and hyposalivation. Ther Clin Risk Manag. 2014; 11:45–51

[53] Biousse V, Skibell BC, Watts RL, Loupe DN, Drews-Botsch C, Newman NJ. Ophthalmologic features of Parkinson's disease. Neurology. 2004; 62(2):177–180

[54] Blumin JH, Pcolinsky DE, Atkins JP. Laryngeal findings in advanced Parkinson's disease. Ann Otol Rhinol Laryngol. 2004; 113(4):253–258

[55] Bakke M, Larsen SL, Lautrup C, Karlsborg M. Orofacial function and oral health in patients with Parkinson's disease. Eur J Oral Sci. 2011; 119(1):27–32

[56] Dirks SJ, Paunovich ED, Terezhalmy GT, Chiodo LK. The Patient with Parkinson's Disease. Quintessence International (Berlin, Germany: 1985). 2003;34(5):379

[57] Bagheri H, Damase-Michel C, Lapeyre-Mestre M, et al. A study of salivary secretion in Parkinson's disease. Clin Neuropharmacol. 1999; 22(4):213–215

[58] Velmurugan MS. Dysgeusia: a review. Asian J Pharm Clin Res. 2013; 6(4):3

[59] Hoover WB. The syndrome of anemia, glossitis, and dysphagia. N Engl J Med. 1935; 213(9):394–398

[60] Gadban H, Gilbey P, Talmon Y, Samet A. Acute edema of the tongue: a life-threatening condition. Ann Otol Rhinol Laryngol. 2003; 112(7):651–653

[61] Shetty S, Pitti V, Satish Babu CL, Surendra Kumar GP, Deepthi BC. Bruxism: a literature review. J Indian Prosthodont Soc. 2010; 10(3):141–148

[62] Clifford T, Finnerty J. The dental awareness and needs of a Parkinson's disease population. Gerodontology. 1995; 12 (12):99–103

[63] Ford ME, Kallen M, Richardson P, et al. Effect of social support on informed consent in older adults with Parkinson disease and their caregivers. J Med Ethics. 2008; 34 (1):41–47

[64] Bair JD, Oppelt TF. Warfarin and ropinirole interaction. Ann Pharmacother. 2001; 35(10):1202–1204

[65] Palareti G, Leali N, Coccheri S, et al. Italian Study on Complications of Oral Anticoagulant Therapy. Bleeding complications of oral anticoagulant treatment: an inception-cohort, prospective collaborative study (ISCOAT). Lancet. 1996; 348 (9025):423–428

[66] Quinonez RB, Kranz AM, Long M, Rozier RG. Care coordination among pediatricians and dentists: a cross-sectional study of opinions of North Carolina dentists. BMC Oral Health. 2014; 14(1):33

[67] Lobbezoo F, Naeije M. Dental implications of some common movement disorders: a concise review. Arch Oral Biol. 2007; 52(4):395–398

[68] Ball MJ, Lillis J. E-health: transforming the physician/patient relationship. Int J Med Inform. 2001; 61(1):1–10

3 Multiple Sclerosis

Haleh Vosgha

Abstract

Multiple sclerosis (MS) is a chronic autoimmune inflammatory disease of the CNS characterized by demyelination of neurons in the brain and spinal cord white matter. Patients with MS disease, which is characterized by the inflammation, demyelination, and scarring (sclerosis) of nerve tissues, initially experience intermittent and eventually chronic neurological dysfunction. Focal damages to the myelin and axons lead to disruption or blocking of nerve signals within the brain and spinal cord, causing a range of debilitating symptoms. MS is the most common cause of neurological disability in young adults, affecting over two million people worldwide. MS usually arises between 15 and 50 years old, with an average onset of 34. Despite ongoing research, the cause of MS is unknown, and its pathophysiology remains poorly understood. Disease-modifying drugs or symptomatic therapies are the current treatment options to help with the management of symptoms and slowing the progression of the disease and relieving specific symptoms. For health practitioners, it is important to comprehensively understand the condition of their patients with MS, especially when they want to perform an invasive procedure. Understanding how to manage, treat, and care for MS patients will allow practitioners to avoid inflicting harm on patients.

Keywords: multiple sclerosis, epidemiology, pathogenesis, oral manifestations, medical management, treatment

3.1 Background of Multiple Sclerosis

Multiple sclerosis (MS) is a chronic autoimmune disease that affects the central nervous system (CNS) and is characterized by the inflammation, demyelination, and scarring (sclerosis: Greek for scarring) of nerve tissues.[1,2,3] Myelin acts as a protective sheath over the nerve tissue. Focal lymphocytic infiltration damages the myelin and axons, which leads to disruption or blocking of nerve signals within the brain and spinal cord, causing a range of debilitating symptoms.[1]

MS is the most common cause of neurological disability in young adults, affecting over 23,000 people in Australia and more than two million people worldwide.[4] Most people are diagnosed between the ages of 20 and 40, and roughly three times as many women have MS as men.[5]

While the earliest descriptions of MS date back to the 14th century, it was French neurologist Jean-Martin Charcot in 1868 who provided the earliest insight into the pathology of MS.[6,7] At a time when many diseases were generalized and grouped as "nervous disorders," Charcot described MS as "*la sclerose en plaques*" and established the Charcot Triad, a set of diagnostic criteria (nystagmus, intention tremor, and scanning speech) to aid in the differentiation between MS and similar diseases of the nervous system.[6,8,9] Through postmortem analysis, Charcot classified the various forms of MS and linked the clinical features of MS with pathological changes in the CNS.[6] Charcot was also the first person to diagnose MS on a living patient.[10]

Since then, research has been focused on achieving a deeper understanding of the mechanisms and processes of MS and on advancing imaging techniques such as MRI.[8] Despite ongoing research on MS, the cause of MS is unknown, and its pathophysiology remains poorly understood.[4] Currently, there is no cure for MS.[3] One leading hypothesis is a combination of genetic disposition in addition to environmental or viral factors.[5] Current treatment options such as disease-modifying drugs or symptomatic therapies help to manage symptoms and slow the progression of the disease or relieve specific symptoms.[5] This chapter aims to discuss multiple sclerosis, and ultimately, the oral complications and management of a patient with MS receiving dental treatment.

3.2 Description of Multiple Sclerosis

MS is an autoimmune inflammatory disease of the CNS. It is characterized by demyelination of neurons in the brain and spinal cord white matter, resulting in initially intermittent and eventually chronic neurological dysfunction.[11,12] MS usually arises between 15 and 50 years, with an average age of onset being 34.[13]

The pathogenesis of MS is complex and involves a range of processes that produce the final sclerotic plaque. MS is initiated by inflammation, followed by demyelination and remyelination. As the disease progresses, astrocytosis and oligodendrocyte depletion occur and toward the final stages, neuronal and axonal loss result.[1] Mature oligodendrocytes are responsible for the synthesis of myelin, a fatty substance that envelopes the axons of neurons within the CNS and is vital to the rapid conduction of nerve signals. Without this myelin sheath, signals are reduced and can even cease, accounting for the neurological dysfunction that is characteristic of MS. Initially in MS, there is transient inflammation, which reduces neuronal conduction and therefore causes episodic dysfunction.[1] However, as the disease evolves, chronic neurodegeneration occurs through the formation of sclerotic plaques in the brain and spinal cord white matter, and this is associated with persistent dysfunction and disability.[1] Thus, the complex pathogenesis of MS accounts for the evolution of symptoms experienced, from episodic to eventually chronic dysfunction (▶ Fig. 3.1).

While the etiology of MS is not completely understood, it is evident that it is multifactorial involving both genetic and environmental factors.[12] Environmental factors such as Epstein-Barr virus, cigarette smoking, and reduced vitamin D levels can interact with and trigger genes in individuals with complex risk profiles, causing an autoimmune response to self-antigens.[11,12,14]

Four forms of MS exist: relapsing remitting MS (RRMS), secondary progressive MS (SPMS), primary progressive MS (PPMS), and progressive relapsing MS (PRMS).[14] RRMS is the most common type and affects 90% of patients.[15] It involves periods of acute neurological disturbances (relapse) that last days to weeks, followed by partial or full recovery.[13,16] About 50% of cases of RRMS progress to SPMS within ten years, which is characterized by worsening of the condition due to neuroaxonal loss without inflammation, independent of relapses.[1,12,13,17] The median age of onset for RRMS and SPMS is 30 years old.[12] PPMS affects 10% of patients, with the median age of onset being 40.[12,15] PPMS is characterized by a gradual progression of disability, without discrete relapses, usually due to spinal motor involvement. PRMS involves a steady progression of the disease with relapses, with or without recovery.[13]

In order to diagnose MS, clinical, radiographical, and laboratory testing evidences (including cerebrospinal fluid analysis and evoked potentials) are utilized. Clinical evidence in terms of the range and severity of symptoms can vary widely among patients and can overlap with other CNS conditions including cognitive impairment, unilateral painful loss of vision, tremor, vertigo, bladder dysfunction, sensory loss, and weakness.[1] Radiographical evidence through magnetic resonance imaging (MRI) aids diagnosis and monitoring of MS. It enables the detection of abnormalities in the white matter of the CNS, thereby indicating the distribution of lesions and aiding the monitoring of new plaques over time.[1] Therefore, the necessity of careful investigations with a complete medical history and physical examination is critical to the correct diagnosis of MS.

While no cure exists for MS, a range of therapies can be used. Medications used include first-line therapies, which stop or slow progression of the disease, while second-line therapies reduce symptoms. Rehabilitation therapies may also be harnessed alongside first- and second-line therapies to improve symptoms.[13,14,15]

Hence, as a multifactorial disease, MS has a complex pathogenesis and requires a range of

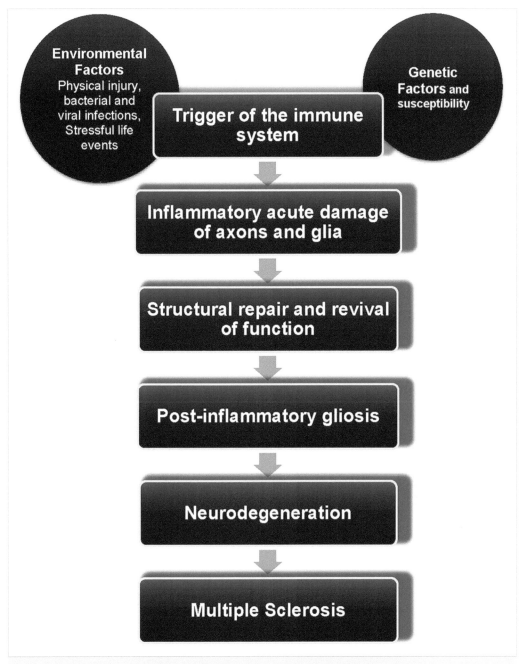

Fig. 3.1 Etiology of multiple sclerosis.

investigations in order to appropriately diagnose and manage the disease. Furthermore, the disease itself has a range of oral and facial manifestations, and many of the medications used in treatment have oral implications, posing an array of considerations for the dental treatment of patients with MS.[13,14,15]

3.3 Epidemiology of Multiple Sclerosis

The most ubiquitous demyelinating disease of the CNS that leads to permanent disability is MS.[18] It has a diverse prevalence throughout the world, and is most commonly seen in developed countries.

3.3.1 Geographical Trends of Multiple Sclerosis

The highest prevalence of MS was found to be in North America (140/100,000 population) and Europe (108/100,000), while the lowest prevalence in East Asia (2.2/100,000 population) and sub-Saharan Africa (2.1/100,000 population).[19] According to the Multiple Sclerosis International Federation, the global median prevalence of the disease has elevated from 2008 to 2013, that is, 30/100,000 to 33/100,000 population, respectively.[19] There are 12,000 new diagnoses of MS per year in the United States alone.[20]

3.3.2 Age- and Sex-related Trends and Mortality Rates of Multiple Sclerosis

Furthermore, the mean age onset of the disease varied from 29 to 33 years old, and the onset was younger in females.[21] A study carried out by Duquette and colleagues have shown that the onset of MS under the age of 10 was 0.3%. They emphasized that childhood MS was more common in females (75.2%).[21]

In addition, the mortality of individuals with the disease was significantly higher than that of the general population when matched for age, gender, race, and ethnicity.[21] The life expectancy of the MS patients was 6 to 14 years lower than that of the healthy population.[19] Also, mortality rates were higher in Caucasian and then subsequently African American, Hispanics, American Indians, and Asian. Caucasian populations had approximately ten times higher mortality rates than Asian populations.[19]

Moreover, due to the increase in the incidence of the MS in women, the MS ratio between male and female has been altered over the past thirty years.[19] From the data obtained by European Database for Multiple Sclerosis system, it is noted that from 1960 to 2005, the gender ratio adjusted for the year of MS onset has increased to 2.45 from 1.60 ($p = 0.017$).[19] The Canadian Collaborative Project on Genetic Susceptibility to MS analyzed the sex ratio (female to male) of MS by year of birth among 27,073 patients born from 1931 to 1980. The ratio was 1.90 for cases born from 1931 to 1935, and increased gradually to 3.21 for those born from 1976 to 1980.[20]

3.3.3 Multiple Sclerosis and Dental Caries

There is a significant association between MS and dental caries. Due to muscle weakness and spasticity and medications, individuals with MS may encounter challenges to maintain basics of oral self-care. MS patients have 2.24 more carious teeth than the general population.[20,22,23]

All in all, the descriptive epidemiological evidence can be utilized for the better understanding of the risk factors and therapeutic implications related to MS.

3.4 Pathogenesis/Etiology of Multiple Sclerosis

The primary cause of damage in MS is thought to be autoimmune inflammation associated with demyelination and phagocytosis in the CNS (▶ Fig. 3.2).[24] Although many studies have suggested that genetic, environmental, and infectious agents may be among the factors influencing the development of MS, the

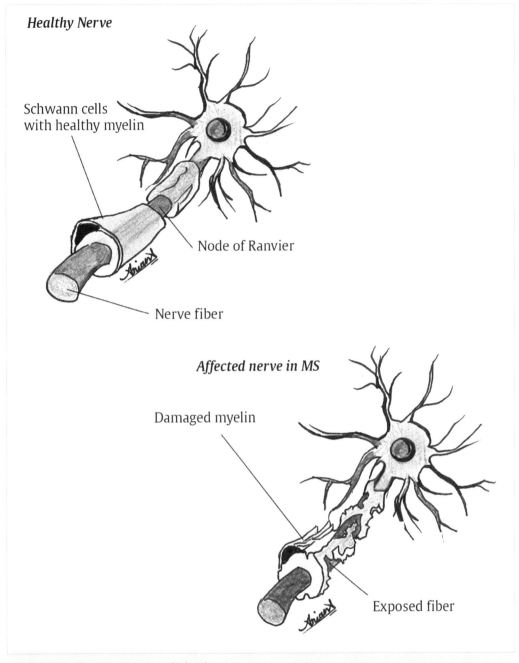

Healthy Nerve

Schwann cells
with healthy myelin

Node of Ranvier

Nerve fiber

Affected nerve in MS

Damaged myelin

Exposed fiber

Fig. 3.2 Demyelination process in multiple sclerosis.

specific elements that start the cause of inflammation are unknown.[24] Demyelination in MS is activated by myelin-reactive T cells in the periphery, which then express adhesion molecules. This allows their entry through the blood–brain barrier (BBB).[14]

Dysregulation of the BBB is one of the earliest cerebrovascular abnormalities seen in MS, as well as the transendothelial migration of activated leukocytes.[25] Breakdown of the BBB allows the immune cells to move across, attacking the myelin around the nerves.[26]

Although the breakdown of BBB is incompletely understood, it suggests involving indirect chemokine/cytokine-dependent leukocyte-mediated injury and direct effects of cytokines/chemokines on the adhesion between the endothelial cells on BBB.[25] During normal immune surveillance, chemokines are responsible for initiating intracellular signaling and guiding the movement of leukocytes through the peripheral tissues.[26] However, during MS chemokines on endothelial cells of BBB are altered, promoting entrance of immune cells.[26]

CD4 T-cells are considered central to initiating the CNS inflammation and are the most used cell type to adoptively transfer encephalomyelitis and most commonly used in experimental model to study the human inflammatory demyelinating disease (experimental autoimmune encephalomyelitis: EAE).[27] However, the array of adaptive immune components (CD8 T-cells and antibody) and innate immune components (microglia/macrophages) reflects the actual extent and specificity of the tissue injuries.[27]

The primary progression of MS is initiated by the innate immune system influencing the effector function of T and B cells.[14] Initiation of the innate immune system involves activation of specific receptors, mainly toll-like receptors (TLRs) in an antigen nonspecific manner through microbial products.[14] TLR-activated dendritic cells (DCs) become semi-mature and produce inhibitory cytokines such as IL-10 or TGF-beta by inducing regulatory T-cells.[14] As maturation of dendritic cells continues, the CD4 T-cells start to differentiate into Th1, Th2, or Th17 phenotypes.[14]

The adaptive response is initiated by the interaction between antigen-presenting cells (APC) and T lymphocytes (T-cells).[14] APC includes B cells, microglia, dendritic cells, and macrophages, which can activate several types of T-cells such as CD4 and CD8. CD4 T-cell, exposed to specific interleukins, polarizes to effector T-cells (Th1, Th2, or Th17).[14] These effector T-cells secrete specific cytokines. Th1 and Th17 secrete proinflammatory cytokines promoting inflammation, while Th2 produce

IL-17, IL-21, IL-22, and IL-26.[14] CD8 cells kill cells, leaving axons exposed and promote vascular permeability, transect axons, activate oligodendrocyte death in the event of MS lesions, and show regulatory function in the progression of MS.[14]

3.5 Genetic Component of Multiple Sclerosis

The neurobiology of MS comprises a complex array of factors, with one of the main components being genetic. The genetic component is suggested by the high incidence of cases in certain ethnic populations and familial aggregation of cases.[28]

The disease is more prevalent in northern European ethnic groups as opposed to Asian or African ethnic groups, irrespective of location. The risk of developing MS increases with a family history of the disease.[29] In European populations, the risk of MS is 0.2%, which increases to 2 to 4% in siblings of MS patients and 30% in monozygotic twins. When studies were done of step-siblings, half-siblings, and adoptees, it was demonstrated that the familial risk was due to genetics and not due to lifestyle conditions.[28]

In the last five years due to the advent of genome-wide studies, the genetic risk factors for MS have increased from 1 to up to 50 various factors.[30] The first genetic risk factor, found in 1970, was the human leukocyte antigen (HLA) region. The HLA region is involved in almost all diseases which are immune related, including MS.[31] HLAs are also known as major histocompatibility complex (MHC) proteins, which are found on the surface of antigen-presenting cells. Each person has a unique set of HLAs, except for identical twins that have the same antigens. The HLAs have a role in cell-to-cell contact during antigen presentation in immune reactions.[31] In MS, the HLA region on chromosome 6p21 has an increased degree of polymorphism, and through DNA-based typing, it was discovered that it was the DRB1*1501 allele.[32] In European population, the frequency of the allele is 3 to 20%. The frequency of the allele has a positive correlation with population risk of MS. Each copy of the allele increases the risk of MS by threefold, making it the strongest genetic indication of MS.[32]

In terms of disease activity, course and severity, and age of onset, MS is considered as a heterogenous disease in a clinical point of view. Studies have shown that there could be genetic implications in these clinical aspects; however, the extent of these implications is relatively unknown.[32] Furthermore, genetic risks that are currently known account for 25% of sibling recurrence risk yet the remaining portion of the risk is unexplained.[30] Although genome-wide research has increased knowledge of the genetic component significantly, the underlying function and clinical mechanisms are yet to be studied.

3.6 Diagnostic Evaluation of Multiple Sclerosis

The identification of MS involves a physician's diagnosis of the condition using their clinical judgment. The diagnosis does not use just one test or is not based on just one clinical feature. It must satisfy certain criteria that have been formalized as the most recent McDonald criteria. According to these criteria, neurologic lesions should show dissemination in space and in time to exclude alternate diagnosis.[11] Initially, these criteria were based on clinical evidence but now these have been updated with the help of MRI and laboratory tests.[11] The diagnosis involves:

- Lesions in two or more separate areas of the CNS including the brain, spinal cord, and optic nerve—indicating dissemination in space (DIS).
- Development of damaged areas being at least one month apart—indicating dissemination in time (DIT).
- Excluding all other possible diagnoses.
- Observing that symptoms occur for more than 24 hours and are experienced as distinct episodes separated by at least one month.
- Magnetic resonance imaging (MRI).
- A spinal tap and testing for oligoclonal bands (OCBs) using cerebrospinal fluid (CSF).[33]

3.6.1 Clinical Symptoms of Multiple Sclerosis

Signs and symptoms of MS usually involve motor, sensory, visual, and autonomic systems (▶ Fig. 3.3) due to the presence of multifocal lesions in the CNS.[1] These vary in an individual depending on the location of the lesion and occur as sudden episodes or as part of a steady progression.[34]

MS is characterized clinically by episodes or relapses of neurological dysfunction.

Usually, individuals experience numbness, weakness, vision loss, gait impairment, incoordination, imbalance, and bladder dysfunction during these episodes. In between the episodes, patients are fairly neurologically stable, but they may experience fatigue or heat sensitivity.[35] As the disease progresses with time, cumulative motor disability and cognitive deficits occur.[36] Characteristic symptoms of MS include the Lhermitte sign, which is an electrical sensation running down the spine or limbs on flexing the neck, and the Uhthoff phenomenon, which is a temporary worsening of symptoms when body temperature rises such as after a hot shower or after exercising.[1]

3.6.2 Radiographical Examination of Multiple Sclerosis

MRI is an important tool to diagnose MS early and to predict its future course. It is a more sensitive way of detecting the clinically silent activity of MS.[36]

It has been studied that 70% of brain lesions and 30% of spinal cord lesions develop without clinical evidence of relapse.[36] MS lesions are usually small and ovoid in shape.[34] Typical sites of MS lesions on MRI include periventricular white matter, juxtacortical white matter, corpus callosum, optic nerve, infratentorial structures (pons, cerebellum, cerebellar peduncles), and the spinal cord.[37]

According to the most recent 2017 McDonald criteria for MS diagnosis, the use of pure imaging can satisfy the criteria of DIT and DIS.[35] Features on an MRI to indicate DIS include more than one T2 lesion (white spots

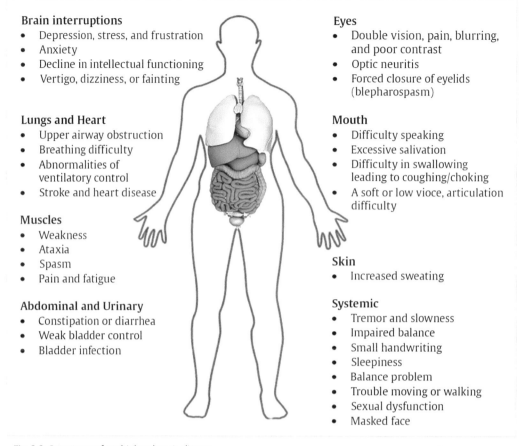

Brain interruptions
- Depression, stress, and frustration
- Anxiety
- Decline in intellectual functioning
- Vertigo, dizziness, or fainting

Lungs and Heart
- Upper airway obstruction
- Breathing difficulty
- Abnormalities of ventilatory control
- Stroke and heart disease

Muscles
- Weakness
- Ataxia
- Spasm
- Pain and fatigue

Abdominal and Urinary
- Constipation or diarrhea
- Weak bladder control
- Bladder infection

Eyes
- Double vision, pain, blurring, and poor contrast
- Optic neuritis
- Forced closure of eyelids (blepharospasm)

Mouth
- Difficulty speaking
- Excessive salivation
- Difficulty in swallowing leading to coughing/choking
- A soft or low vioce, articulation difficulty

Skin
- Increased sweating

Systemic
- Tremor and slowness
- Impaired balance
- Small handwriting
- Sleepiness
- Balance problem
- Trouble moving or walking
- Sexual dysfunction
- Masked face

Fig. 3.3 Symptoms of multiple sclerosis disease.

seen in an MRI scan that indicate inflammation or permanent scarring) in at least two of the typical sites mentioned above. Features to indicate DIT include asymptomatic lesions presenting simultaneously at any time, or one or more new T2 lesion on follow-up MRI at any time.[34]

3.6.3 Laboratory Testing of Multiple Sclerosis

Paraclinical studies to diagnose MS include CSF analysis and evoked potential testing.

3.6.4 CSF Analysis

Immunoglobulin G (IgG) OCBs are unique to the CSF. The detection of OCBs in the CSF suggests inflammation within, which corresponds to the nature of MS.[38] In more than 90% of patients, CSF analysis showed increased concentrations of IgG and at least two OCBs.[35] OCB testing must be done within 72 hours of a lumbar puncture to obtain the CSF serum.[36]

3.6.5 Evoked Potentials

Evoked potentials are used to display delayed conduction in CNS sensory pathways when other methods of diagnosis are insufficient to provide objective evidence of a multifocal disease. Afferent visual pathways, auditory pathways, and dorsal-column sensory pathways, including nerves that innervate upper and lower extremities, are evaluated by evoked potentials. Slowed conduction times, especially if asymmetric, indicate MS.[35,39]

3.6.6 Medical History of Multiple Sclerosis

The history of MS patients is usually of having episodes of typical demyelinating events separated by time, in terms of disease course, and space, in terms of anatomic locations. The first clinical episode indicative of MS is called the clinically isolated syndrome (CIS).[34] Patients with CIS, particularly those with brain lesions consistent with MS on MRI, have high chances of developing MS in the future.[40] CIS patients mostly presented with symptoms such as optic neuritis (pain on eye movement, blurred vision), motor or sensory deficits, brainstem syndrome involving blurred or double vision, and multifocal abnormalities, which usually involve the spinal cord.[37]

3.6.7 Physical Examination of Multiple Sclerosis

A thorough physical examination is important to determine deficits in MS. All systems must be taken into account, including cognition, motor, sensory, musculoskeletal, reflexes, coordination, vision, gait, and skin.[41] Individuals may show a variety of abnormal physical outcomes that may change by the next examination. This depends on the pattern of disease and whether the patient is experiencing relapses.[41] Standard outcomes include localized weakness, focal sensory disruption, hyperactive reflexes with clonus (involuntary muscle spasms) in ankles, increased stiffness in extremities, poor coordination, Lhermitte sign, and wide-based gait with being unable to tandem walk. An ophthalmologic examination is required to address optic neuritis, which involves the sensory visual pathway causing acute unilateral loss of visual acuity, deficits in color and contrast sensitivity, visual field changes, and pain.[41]

3.7 Medical Management and Treatment of Multiple Sclerosis

MS is a chronic, progressive relapsing disorder that requires multidisciplinary therapies and coordinated care between patient, doctors, and rehabilitation specialists.[42] At present, there is, unfortunately, no curative treatment for MS. There are two lines of medications for management of MS: first-line therapies, including steroids and immunosuppressants, that halt or slow disease progression and reduce the frequency and severity of relapse episodes; and second-line therapies that aim to reduce the symptoms of disease.[43] Rehabilitation therapies may also be integrated with medications to improve symptoms.[44]

3.7.1 First-line Disease-modifying Therapies

First-line therapies aim to halt or slow disease progression by targeting the underlying immunological abnormality. Corticosteroid, anti-inflammatory, and immunosuppressive therapies are commonly used.

Corticosteroid, or simply, steroid therapies, such as methylprednisolone and prednisone, treat acute relapses of MS.[43] Steroid therapies act on the immune response to regulate cytokine and chemokine secretions, thereby inducing the apoptosis and reducing activation of T-cells. They have also been found to decrease levels of metalloproteinases and tissue inhibitors of metalloproteinases in cerebrospinal fluid, reduce numbers of adhesion molecules, and reduce interference with the BBB.[44] Short-term high doses of methylprednisolone increased the speed of recovery from relapses but did not alter the degree of recovery, the onset of relapses, or the long-term prognosis of the disease. Methylprednisolone may also be administered orally or intravenously, and there are minimal differences with equivalent doses with either route of administration. Intravenous administration is preferred over oral administration as studies show evidence of a higher correlation with side effects, such as dyspepsia, emotional instability, hypertension, or osteoporosis with oral administration.[45]

Anti-inflammatory or immunosuppressive therapies may also be administered to manage MS. Anti-inflammatory immunosuppressive medications prescribed include beta-interferon, copolymer-1, methotrexate, glatiramer acetate, teriflunomide, natalizumab, alemtuzumab, mitoxantrone, fingolimod, and dimethyl fumarate.[43,46]

Beta-interferon therapy is a common line of anti-inflammatory therapy that reduces the number and size of demyelinating lesions.[43] Interferon beta may be administered intramuscularly or subcutaneously, although the latter is quite expensive. The subcutaneous administration has been shown to reduce the frequency of relapse episodes.[42] Interferon beta is a naturally occurring polypeptide produced by fibroblasts. It has anti-inflammatory actions, is the form of inhibition of T-cell proliferation, changes cytokines to be anti-inflammatory, and reduces migration of inflammatory cells across the BBB. However, flulike symptoms are common side effects upon commencement of interferon beta medication, including aches, pain, fever, chills, and headaches; also, liver enzymes may be elevated, and bone marrow function may be depressed.[46]

While there is no curative treatment available for MS, corticosteroid and immunosuppressive therapies aid the delay of disease progression and recovery following relapses.

3.7.2 Second-line Symptomatic Therapies

Disease-modifying therapies do not always relieve the symptoms associated with MS. Symptoms include mood disorders/depression, cognitive dysfunction, optic neuritis, diplopia, paresthesia, tremor, spasticity, and muscle weakness.[43] Symptomatic therapies are given in conjunction with first-line therapies to alleviate such symptoms and improve quality of life.

Antidepressants may be prescribed to alleviate mood disorders, depression, and feelings of euphoria or indifference. Cognitive dysfunction caused by demyelination is treated with cognitive therapy, although this is not very effective. Optic neuritis, or inflammation of the optic nerve, may be relieved with steroid medications, including those given as first-line

therapy for MS. Diplopia, or double vision, can be simply corrected by covering one eye. Anticonvulsants are given to relieve paresthesia. Muscle relaxants, such as baclofen, benzodiazepine, or dantrolene, are commonly administered to reduce pain caused by spastic paralysis, bladder dysfunction, or tremors. Evidence shows that weakness and loss of sensation can be reversed with the potassium channel blocker, 4-aminopyridine, which allows partially demyelinated axons to conduct impulses again and thus restore function.[43]

Second-line therapies do not target the underlying cause of MS; however, they may be implemented to produce symptomatic relief and improve the patient's quality of life.

3.7.3 Rehabilitation Therapies of Multiple Sclerosis

Multidisciplinary rehabilitation, including physiotherapy, occupational therapy, psychology, and psychiatry, in combination with medicinal lines of therapy provides further symptomatic relief.[44] Motor and cognitive tests showed improvements to disability, quality of life, and severity of relapses when rehabilitation is utilized in combination with first- and second-line therapies. Beneficial effects of rehabilitation are also evidenced in children diagnosed with MS. These children often suffer from poor concentration, which can manifest as risk-taking behavior, substance abuse, and school and family dysfunction. This warrants intervention from psychologists, social workers, and special needs education.[47]

Medical management of MS involves disease-modifying drugs, which target the underlying cause of the disease, and symptomatic therapies to relieve associated symptoms of MS. Medicinal intervention may be complemented by rehabilitative therapies.

3.8 Management of a Dental Patient with Multiple Sclerosis

Oral and facial manifestations can occur with MS and its medications, and the dentist may be the first to identify these. Such manifestations need to be appropriately managed by the dentist, and treatment tailored to the severity and nature of disease progression. Furthermore, a certain number of drugs currently prescribed by dentists may interact with medications prescribed for MS, so awareness of contraindications and precautions and liaising with specialists and doctors is critical.

3.8.1 Oral and Facial Manifestations of Multiple Sclerosis

Oral and facial manifestations that may be associated with MS include trigeminal neuralgia, trigeminal sensory paresthesia, facial palsy, dysphagia, temporomandibular joint disorders, and optic neuritis. Dentists and other oral health professionals may be the first to identify the symptoms of these manifestations, which worsen with MS disease progression.[48]

Trigeminal neuralgia is caused by sclerotic plaque formation along the course of the trigeminal nerve.[22] This causes pain that may be provoked by mastication, touching the cheek, or tooth-brushing.[48,49] Trigeminal sensory paresthesia is characterized by numbness of the lower lip and chin, and may or may not have associated pain. Numbness may be provoked by local trauma, odontogenic lesions, and neoplasms of the jaw, so it is important that dentists identify these issues early to prevent paresthesia.[49] Facial palsy is an early orofacial manifestation of MS; thus, it may act as an indicator of undiagnosed MS. Dysphagia may develop in mildly impaired MS and progressively worsen with progression of MS.[50] Of particular importance to dentistry is temporomandibular joint disorder, which has been linked to MS due to cerebellar ataxia, fatigue of masticatory muscles, and lack of coordination of mandibular movement.[51] As mentioned earlier, optic neuritis or inflammation of the optic nerve due to demyelination can also occur, leading to partial, transient loss of vision; however, this is alleviated with steroid therapies administered for MS.

Tremors, compromised manual dexterity, chronic pain, and loss of self-motivation that may be associated with MS can affect a patient's oral hygiene[42]; these factors should be taken into consideration when formulating a dental treatment plan. MS patients may be at higher risk of developing gingivitis and periodontitis due to increased susceptibility to plaque accumulation from loss of manual dexterity and increased risk with certain medications administered, such as interferon beta.[22] Such medications may also cause gingival hyperplasia, mucositis/ulcerative stomatitis, dysgeusia, candidiasis, angular cheilitis, herpes simplex virus infections, or xerostomia, and even certain forms of cancer (lymphoma, squamous cell carcinoma) in some patients who have been on long-term immunosuppressive therapy.[22,49]

Early diagnosis by dentists may contribute to the diagnosis of MS, or relief or prevention of these symptoms, where possible.

3.9 Oral Medicine Aspects of Multiple Sclerosis

3.9.1 Drug–Drug Interactions

Medications to manage MS can interact with medications used in dentistry, and these interactions (▶ Table 3.1) can alter drug metabolism, or even cause cytotoxicity and hepatotoxicity.[22]

The cardinal signs of inflammation are masked by steroid or anti-inflammatory medications. This makes difficult to differentiate chronic pain associated with MS from pain associated with dental infection. Nonsteroidal anti-inflammatories, aspirin, acetaminophen, and erythromycin are common medications prescribed by dentists for pain relief. Precautions should be taken when prescribing nonsteroidal anti-inflammatory medications or aspirin to MS patients on steroid therapy, as there is a significant elevation in the risk of gastric ulcers when these medications are taken in combination.[49] Nonsteroidal anti-inflammatories and aspirin significantly increase the cytotoxicity of methotrexate by increasing the amount of free methotrexate available, so these drugs should be used very prudently on patients taking methotrexate.[49]

Table 3.1 Common oral medications administered for the management of multiple sclerosis, their mechanisms of action and adverse effects

Generic name	Trade name	Mechanism of action	Adverse systemic reactions
Prednisone	Deltasone	Belongs to a class of drugs known as corticosteroids.[52] It is taken via the mouth, usually directed by the doctor once a day. Prednisone can be seen as a white to practically white, odorless, crystalline powder, and is available in five strengths: 2.5 mg, 5 mg, 10 mg, 20 mg, and 50 mg.[52] Dosage amounts are specified to each patient's need and response of the patient. Quantitatively, MS patients will have 200 mg of prednisone for a week for results to show up effective.[52]	Side effects of the medication include fluid and electrolyte disturbances[53]: sodium retention, fluid retention, congestive heart failure in susceptible patients, potassium loss, hypokalemic alkalosis, and hypertension. Musculoskeletal[53]: muscle weakness, steroid myopathy, loss of muscle mass, osteoporosis, muscle pain, etc. Dermatologic[53]: impaired wound healing, thin fragile skin, etc. Neurological[53]: headaches, vertigo, convulsions. In addition, it can cause urticarial and other allergic, anaphylactic, or hypersensitivity reactions.
Methylprednisolone (oral)	Medrol	Medrol tablets consist of methylprednisolone, a glucocorticoid.[54] This means both naturally occurring and synthetic, thus easily absorbed by the gastrointestinal tract. They help control the severity of any MS attacks, via reducing the inflammation at the site of infection.[54] It also assists in the acute exacerbations of MS. Medrol tablets come in five dosages of 2 mg, 4 mg, 8 mg, 16 mg, and 32 mg.[54]	Possible side effects of Medrol include gastrointestinal problems[55]: peptic ulcer with possible perforation and hemorrhage, pancreatitis, abdominal distention, ulcerative esophagitis, increases in alanine transaminase (usually seen with any corticosteroid treatment). Dermatologic side effects include[55]: impaired wound healing, increased sweating, and thin fragile skin. Metabolic disturbances include negative nitrogen balance due to protein catabolism.[55]
Fingolimod	Gilenya	Fingolimod helps to reduce relapse rate, decrease the frequency of acute attacks. This delays the accumulation of physical disability.[56] It is a 1-phosphate receptor modulator, acting to reduce the number of lymphocytes (white blood cells) in the peripheral blood.[56] It is usually administered in a dose of 0.5 mg once a day orally. The prescription usually can last for a period of 12 months.[56]	Common side effects include headaches, high blood pressure, blurred vision, influenza, diarrhea, back pain, increase in liver enzymes, and cough.[56] Fingolimod also causes slowing of the heartbeat, which is why with the first dose patients must have their heart rate monitored for the first 6 hours.[56] Blurred vision is caused by macular retinal edema, meaning eye problems.[56]
Teriflunomide	Aubagio	Teriflunomide acts as an oral pyrimidine synthesis inhibitor, which can be seen as a white to almost white powder.[57] Aubagio contains 7 mg to 14 mg of teriflunomide along with other inactive ingredients (lactose monohydrate, corn starch, hydroxypropylcellulose, microcrystalline cellulose, sodium starch glycolate, and magnesium stearate).[57] The tablets are film-coated, allowing the medication to be administrated orally. It is taken once daily, to help reduce relapse rate.[57]	Side effects of teriflunomide include risk of liver damage, hair loss or thinning of hair, nausea, diarrhea, influenza, burning or prickly feeling in skin, and/or numbness or tingling in limbs.[57] Patients that consume Aubagio should therefore be cautious of hepatotoxicity and keep watch of their plasma concentrations. Aubagio has the potential to cause fetal harm if administered during pregnancy.[57] Teratogenicity could occur, and so Aubagio is contraindicated for use in pregnant women.[57]
Dimethyl fumarate	Tecfidera	Tecfidera works as a delayed-release capsule, which contains 120 mg or 240 mg of dimethyl fumarate in the form of an off-white powder.[58] The hard gelatin delayed-release capsules also contain inactive ingredients of microcrystalline cellulose, silicified microcrystalline cellulose.[58] It is given in 120 mg doses to be taken twice a day orally.[58]	With supplements of Tecfidera, possible adverse reactions that can occur are anaphylaxis and angioedema, progressive multifocal leukoencephalopathy, lymphopenia, liver injury, and flushing.[58] There have also been studies to indicate that Tecfidera causes gastrointestinal events like nausea, vomiting, diarrhea, abdominal pain, and dyspepsia.[58]

Drug interactions between acetaminophen prescribed by dentists for pain relief and anticonvulsants, phenytoin or carbamazepine, can lead to hepatotoxicity through the accumulation of derivatives of acetaminophen. Furthermore, the antibiotic, erythromycin, diminishes the clearance of phenytoin and carbamazepine, thereby increasing their toxicity.[22]

Interactions between drugs prescribed in dentistry and those administered to patients with MS should be checked for safety, toxicity, contraindications, and precautions before administration and used prudently.

3.9.2 Prior to and during Dental Treatment

Individuals who have MS have an increased risk of gingivitis and periodontitis and dental caries due to the patients' reduced immune response and the physical effects of the disease.[59] This should be considered when planning the dental treatment and oral hygiene procedures for an MS patient. As chronic periodontitis involves inflammation and systemic inflammation is a trigger for MS, basic periodontal treatment is beneficial.[22] This treatment includes removal of supragingival and subgingival plaque and calculus, which reduced the overall inflammatory response in the body. MS patients have more decay, restored or missing teeth, and more severe periodontal disease than those without MS.[59]

Physical disability is a barrier to self-care in MS patients as their manual dexterity is affected.[60] In these circumstances, an electric toothbrush may be useful. A caregiver can also provide physical support whilst the patient performs oral hygiene practices. Flossing can be done sitting down and, in the morning, when the patient is not so tired. If the patient is unable to floss by themselves, they may be assisted by their caregiver. If there is a lack of oral hygiene care, more frequent dental appointments can be scheduled to maintain oral hygiene. Xerostomia is dryness of the oral cavity and can occur as a side effect of the medication that individuals with MS use.[61] This should be considered when undertaking dental treatment and it may be recommended for an individual to chew xylitol—a sugar-free chewing gum.

When treating patients with MS, short appointments in the morning are preferable. Treatment plans should be adapted if the patient experiences pain, fatigue, difficulty swallowing, spasticity, or paralysis.[62] Patients should be able to make their preferences known regarding oral care; however, in more advanced stages, a caregiver may have to make some decisions on behalf of the patient.[22] Individuals with mild MS are much more likely to attend dental appointments than those with severe symptoms. Patients may experience barriers such as access to the dental office, waiting room, parking, and bathrooms. Oral health professionals should be considerate of these barriers and promote safety for patients by keeping hallways clear, noticing changes in the patient's stride, mobility, and dexterity, being flexible in appointment targets, helping the patient to the restroom or door, and scheduling appointments in the dental chair as opposed to a reception.[59]

3.10 Coordination of Care between Dentist and Physician

Multiple sclerosis and the medications prescribed for its management may have several oral and facial manifestations, which require coordinated care between the patient, dentists, and physicians.

MS is known to have a widespread effect on the body as it affects the nerves of the CNS. Therefore, the effects of MS can spread to the orofacial region and lead to various complications. As aforementioned, the main manifestations that are of importance to a dentist include facial palsy, trigeminal neuralgia, and sensory neuropathy of the trigeminal nerve.[49] Medications that are taken by MS patients can also affect their oral health negatively by increasing their susceptibility to dental diseases. Thus, there needs to be communication between the dentist and physician of MS patients in order for early diagnosis and management of these potential oral and facial manifestations.

Treatment of MS usually involves the use of corticosteroids, immunosuppressors, interferons, and anticonvulsants.[63] Corticosteroids also make MS patients at greater risk of adrenal atrophy with dental treatment, which can lead to an adrenal crisis (emesis, shock, diarrhea, abdominal pain, even fatal), so dentists should proceed with caution. As previously mentioned, immunosuppressants, such as methotrexate, and interferons can lead to neutropenia and anemia. Hence, patients undergoing surgical procedures should be placed on prophylactic antibiotics as they are more susceptible to bacterial infections.[64] Furthermore, aspirin and nonsteroidal anti-inflammatories frequently prescribed by dentists can negatively interact with methotrexate to increase its cytotoxicity, and thus should be administered cautiously. Evidently, it is important that if steroids, immunosuppressants, and interferons are implemented by physicians, this should be communicated to the patient's dentist. Anticonvulsants (e.g., carbamazepine, phenytoin) are also commonly prescribed by physicians to control the pain of trigeminal neuralgia.[63] Also, the anticonvulsant carbamazepine can cause bone marrow suppression and lead to anemia and thrombocytopenia.[65] Therefore, the use of anticonvulsants must be communicated to the dentist to safely plan their treatment of the patient's oral health.

The severity of the patient's condition and associated pain should also be comprehensively communicated to the dentist. This information is essential in formatting an appropriate dental course of care and assessing the probability of a successful prognosis. Pain levels, pain frequency, and types of pain, including paresthesia, dysesthesia, and hyperesthesia, should also be discussed between dentist and physician. An understanding of the patient's pain levels and frequency will aid in preventing any unnecessary harm to the patient and also provide information on treatment plans and medication to avoid with specific patients.

It can be concluded that MS is a very important neurological disease that can cause serious implications for patients who attain it. There have been various studies conducted on MS and they have established that MS patients require special consideration and treatment as they can be susceptible to harmful side effects should they be exposed to certain hazardous factors. As a dentist, it is highly important to comprehensively understand the condition of MS patients, as the profession demands clinicians to work in close proximity of patients and frequently participate in invasive procedures. Understanding how to manage, treat, and care for MS patients will allow practitioners to avoid inflicting harm on patients.

References

[1] Compston A, Coles A. Multiple sclerosis. Lancet. 2008; 372 (9648):1502–1517
[2] Hemmer B, Cepok S, Nessler S, Sommer N. Pathogenesis of multiple sclerosis: an update on immunology. Curr Opin Neurol. 2002; 15(3):227–231
[3] Hellings N, Raus J, Stinissen P. Insights into the immunopathogenesis of multiple sclerosis. Immunol Res. 2002; 25(1): 27–51
[4] Rolak LA. Multiple sclerosis: it's not the disease you thought it was. Clin Med Res. 2003; 1(1):57–60
[5] Pietrangelo A, Higuera V. Multiple Sclerosis by the Numbers: Facts, Statistics, and You: Healthline; 2017. Available at: http://www.healthline.com/health/multiple-sclerosis/facts-statistics-infographic. Accessed May 16, 2019
[6] Kumar DR, Aslinia F, Yale SH, Mazza JJ. Jean-Martin Charcot: the father of neurology. Clin Med Res. 2011; 9(1):46–49
[7] Lublin F. History of modern multiple sclerosis therapy. J Neurol. 2005; 252 Suppl 3:iii3–iii9
[8] Murray TJ. The history of multiple sclerosis: the changing frame of the disease over the centuries. J Neurol Sci. 2009; 277 Suppl 1:S3–S8
[9] Poser CM, Brinar VV. Diagnostic criteria for multiple sclerosis. Clin Neurol Neurosurg. 2001; 103(1):1–11
[10] Pearce JM. Historical descriptions of multiple sclerosis. Eur Neurol. 2005; 54(1):49–53
[11] Nylander A, Hafler DA. Multiple sclerosis. J Clin Invest. 2012; 122(4):1180–1188
[12] McKay KA, Kwan V, Duggan T, Tremlett H. Risk factors associated with the onset of relapsing-remitting and primary progressive multiple sclerosis: a systematic review. BioMed Res Int. 2015; 2015:817238
[13] Wilson N. Primary Care: Oral disease modifying therapies for multiple sclerosis. AJP. Australas J Pharm. 2017; 98(1163):70–73

[14] Loma I, Heyman R. Multiple sclerosis: pathogenesis and treatment. Curr Neuropharmacol. 2011; 9(3):409–416

[15] Raffel J, Wakerley B, Nicholas R. Multiple sclerosis. Medicine. 2016; 44(9):537–541

[16] Gray O, Rensel M. Fast Facts: Multiple Sclerosis. 4th ed. Basel, Switzerland :Health Press Limited; 2016:144

[17] Courtney AM, Treadaway K, Remington G, Frohman E. Multiple sclerosis. Med Clin North Am. 2009; 93(2):451–476, ix–x

[18] Koch-Henriksen N, Sørensen PS. The changing demographic pattern of multiple sclerosis epidemiology. Lancet Neurol. 2010; 9(5):520–532

[19] Leray E, Moreau T, Fromont A, Edan G. Epidemiology of multiple sclerosis. Rev Neurol (Paris). 2016; 172(1):3–13

[20] Alonso A, Hernán MA. Temporal trends in the incidence of multiple sclerosis: a systematic review. Neurology. 2008; 71 (2):129–135

[21] Ramagopalan SV, Sadovnick AD. Epidemiology of multiple sclerosis. Neurol Clin. 2011; 29(2):207–217

[22] Elemek E, Almas K. Multiple sclerosis and oral health: an update. N Y State Dent J. 2013; 79(3):16–21

[23] Santa Eulalia-Troisfontaines E, Martínez-Pérez EM, Miegimolle-Herrero M, Planells-Del Pozo P. Oral health status of a population with multiple sclerosis. Med Oral Patol Oral Cir Bucal. 2012; 17(2):e223–e227

[24] McFarland HF, Martin R. Multiple sclerosis: a complicated picture of autoimmunity. Nat Immunol. 2007; 8(9):913–919

[25] Minagar A, Alexander JS. Blood-brain barrier disruption in multiple sclerosis. Mult Scler. 2003; 9(6):540–549

[26] Holman DW, Klein RS, Ransohoff RM. The blood-brain barrier, chemokines and multiple sclerosis. Biochim Biophys Acta. 2011; 1812(2):220–230

[27] Prat A, Antel J. Pathogenesis of multiple sclerosis. Curr Opin Neurol. 2005; 18(3):225–230

[28] Gourraud PA, Harbo HF, Hauser SL, Baranzini SE. The genetics of multiple sclerosis: an up-to-date review. Immunol Rev. 2012; 248(1):87–103

[29] Haines JL, Ter-Minassian M, Bazyk A, et al. The Multiple Sclerosis Genetics Group. A complete genomic screen for multiple sclerosis underscores a role for the major histocompatibility complex. Nat Genet. 1996; 13(4):469–471

[30] Mechelli R, Annibali V, Ristori G, Vittori D, Coarelli G, Salvetti M. Multiple sclerosis etiology: beyond genes and environment. Expert Rev Clin Immunol. 2010; 6(3):481–490

[31] Damjanov I. Pathology for the Health Professions. 4th ed. St Louis: Saunders; 2012

[32] Goris A, Pauwels I, Dubois B. Progress in multiple sclerosis genetics. Curr Genomics. 2012; 13(8):646–663

[33] Goldenberg MM. Multiple sclerosis review. P&T. 2012; 37(3): 175–184

[34] Milo R, Miller A. Revised diagnostic criteria of multiple sclerosis. Autoimmun Rev. 2014; 13(4–5):518–524

[35] Thompson AJ, Banwell BL, Barkhof F, et al. Diagnosis of multiple sclerosis: 2017 revisions of the McDonald criteria. Lancet Neurol. 2018 Feb; 17(2):162–173. doi:10.1016/S1474-4422 (17)30470-2

[36] Karussis D. The diagnosis of multiple sclerosis and the various related demyelinating syndromes: a critical review. J Autoimmun. 2014; 48–49:134–142

[37] Tsang BK, Macdonell R. Multiple sclerosis- diagnosis, management and prognosis. Aust Fam Physician. 2011; 40(12): 948–955

[38] Álvarez-Cermeño JC, Villar LM. Multiple sclerosis: oligoclonal bands–a useful tool to avoid MS misdiagnosis. Nat Rev Neurol. 2013; 9(6):303–304

[39] Katz Sand IB, Lublin FD. Diagnosis and differential diagnosis of multiple sclerosis. Continuum (N Y). 2013; 19:922–943

[40] Katz Sand I. Classification, diagnosis, and differential diagnosis of multiple sclerosis. Curr Opin Neurol. 2015; 28(3):193–205

[41] Luzzio C. Multiple Sclerosis Clinical Presentation Medscape 2017. https://emedicine.medscape.com/article/1146199-clinical. Updated May 23, 2019. Accessed May 25, 2019

[42] Scully C, Bain S, Hamburger J. Common Medical Conditions: A Guide for the Dental Team: John Wiley & Sons; 2009

[43] Young RR. Diagnosis and medical management of multiple sclerosis. J Spinal Cord Med. 1998; 21(2):109–112

[44] Nedeljkovic U, Dackovic J, Tepavcevic D, et al. Multidisciplinary rehabilitation and steroids in the management of multiple sclerosis relapses: a randomised controlled trial. Arch Med Sci. 2014; 2:380–389

[45] Myhr KM, Mellgren SI. Corticosteroids in the treatment of multiple sclerosis. Acta Neurol Scand Suppl. 2009; 120(189): 73–80

[46] Torkildsen Ø, Myhr KM, Bø L. Disease-modifying treatments for multiple sclerosis - a review of approved medications. Eur J Neurol. 2016; 23 Suppl 1:18–27

[47] Govender R. Guideline for the diagnosis and management of multiple sclerosis in children. S Afr Med J. 2013; 103(9) Suppl 3:692–695

[48] Lassemi E, Sahraian M, Motamedi M, Valayi M, Moradi N, Lasemi R. Oral and facial manifestations of patients with multiple sclerosis. Dentistry. 2014; 4(2)

[49] Chemaly D, Lefrançois A, Pérusse R. Oral and maxillofacial manifestations of multiple sclerosis. J Can Dent Assoc. 2000; 66(11):600–605

[50] De Pauw A, Dejaeger E, D'hooghe B, Carton H. Dysphagia in multiple sclerosis. Clin Neurol Neurosurg. 2002; 104(4):345–351

[51] Carvalho L, Matta A, Nascimento O. Temporomandibular disorders (TMD) and multiple sclerosis (MS) (P1.120). Neurology. 2015; 84(14) Suppl

[52] Perumal JS, Caon C, Hreha S, et al. Oral prednisone taper following intravenous steroids fails to improve disability or recovery from relapses in multiple sclerosis. Eur J Neurol. 2008; 15(7):677–680

[53] Chrousos GA, Kattah JC, Beck RW, Cleary PA. Side effects of glucocorticoid treatment. Experience of the Optic Neuritis Treatment Trial. JAMA. 1993; 269(16):2110–2112

[54] Sloka JS, Stefanelli M. The mechanism of action of methylprednisolone in the treatment of multiple sclerosis. Mult Scler. 2005; 11(4):425–432

[55] Alam SM, Kyriakides T, Lawden M, Newman PK. Methylprednisolone in multiple sclerosis: a comparison of oral with intravenous therapy at equivalent high dose. J Neurol Neurosurg Psychiatry. 1993; 56(11):1219–1220

[56] Jeffrey A, Cohen FB. Oral fingolimod or intramuscular interferon for relapsing multiple sclerosis. N Engl J Med. 2010; 2010(362):402–415

[57] Confavreux C, Li DK, Freedman MS, et al. Teriflunomide Multiple Sclerosis Trial Group. Long-term follow-up of a phase 2 study of oral teriflunomide in relapsing multiple sclerosis: safety and efficacy results up to 8.5 years. Mult Scler. 2012; 18(9):1278–1289

[58] Bomprezzi R. Dimethyl fumarate in the treatment of relapsing-remitting multiple sclerosis: an overview. Ther Adv Neurol Disorder. 2015; 8(1):20–30

[59] Schroeder K, Gruenlian J. Oral health risks of multiple sclerosis. Decisions in Dentistry. 2017; 3(2):40–43

[60] Scully C. Mouth ulcers and other causes of orofacial soreness and pain. West J Med. 2001; 174(6):421–424

[61] Fiske J, Griffiths J, Thompson S. Multiple sclerosis and oral care. Dent Update. 2002; 29(6):273–283

[62] Fischer DJ, Epstein JB, Klasser G. Multiple sclerosis: an update for oral health care providers. Oral Surg Oral Med Oral Pathol Oral Radiol Endod. 2009; 108(3):318–327

[63] DiPiro J, Talbert R, Yee G, Matzke G, Wells B, Posey M. Pharmacotherapy: A Pathophysiologic Approach. 3rd ed. New York: Appleton & Lange; 1997

[64] Perusse R. Désordres Systémiques: Planifications des soins Dentaires. 1st ed. Canada: The Press of Laval University; 1996

[65] Canadian Pharmacists Association. Compendium of Pharmaceuticals and Specialties. 34th ed. Toronto: Canadian Pharmacists Association; 1999

4 Amyotrophic Lateral Sclerosis

Armin Ariana

Abstract

Amyotrophic lateral sclerosis (ALS) is the most common fatal progressive neurodegenerative disease and has significant effects on functionality, independency, and overall quality of life. It is a non-cell-autonomous disease that targets the motor neurons and the surrounding glia in the brainstem, corticospinal tract, and spinal anterior horn. Characterized by limb weakness, falls, communication, and swallowing difficulties to cognitive and behavioral changes, the severity and range of symptoms differ from case to case. Despite the heterogeneous presentation of symptoms, most cases result in death by respiratory failure, as the lungs and their supporting muscles simply loose optimal vitality to perform their proper function. ALS has an unknown etiology; therefore, its diagnosis becomes a challenge and the commencement of management can be belated. Currently with no cure, symptomatic alleviation is utilized; however, several therapeutic drugs are currently being tested in clinical trials. Modifications to procedural treatment are recommended to ensure the comfort and protection of ALS patients; and multidisciplinary clinical coordination is essential for optimizing health care delivery, increasing survival rate, and enhancing the quality of life of ALS patients.

Keywords: amyotrophic lateral sclerosis, epidemiology, pathogenesis, oral manifestations, medical management, treatment

microgliosis directly contributes to neurodegeneration.[3] It is characterized by progressive degeneration of the brainstem, corticospinal tract, and spinal anterior horn.[4]

ALS was first described by both Aran and Cruveilhier in 1848 and 1853, respectively. It was not until 1869 that Charles Charcot defined and identified the disease we now know as ALS.[1] Several years later, Charcot stated that ALS was not hereditary; however, in the 1950s Kurland and Mulder established a genetic link to approximately 10% of cases.[1] ALS became a household name in 1939 when American baseball player Lou Gehrig was diagnosed with the disease at 36 years old, putting an end to his illustrious career. Since this time, ALS was also synonymously known as Lou Gehrig disease.[1]

ALS sufferers have an extremely poor prognosis, with no cure or viable treatment available. The median survival time postdiagnosis is 3 years, while only 5% can expect to survive 10 years.[5,6] This poor prognosis is thought to be, in some parts, due to delays in commencement of therapeutic treatments. The average time to commit to a diagnosis is 1 year.[6] A more noteworthy delay in treatment is the physical manifestations experienced by patients, thought to be considerably downstream to the pathological changes that occur. This leaves an unanswered question: Would early diagnosis and intervention halt the progression or even lead to a cure of ALS?[6]

4.1 Background of Amyotrophic Lateral Sclerosis

Amyotrophic lateral sclerosis (ALS) is a progressive disorder and the most common fatal neurodegenerative disease.[1] It is a non–cell-autonomous disease that targets the motor neurons and the surrounding glia.[2] Recent studies showed microglia was implicated in the initiation of ALS, wherein the presence of

4.2 Description of Amyotrophic Lateral Sclerosis

The characteristic symptoms of ALS include limb weakness, falls, communication, and swallowing difficulties to cognitive and behavioral changes.[7,8] The severity and range of symptoms differ from case to case.[7] Despite this heterogeneous presentation of symptoms, most cases result in death by respiratory failure,[7] as the lungs and their supporting muscles simply loose optimal vitality to perform their proper function.[9]

The onset of symptoms is categorized into bulbar onset (the symptom first noticed is slurred speech) and limb onset (the symptom first noticed is a weakness in the upper or lower limbs).[1] Some phenotypes have only upper or lower motor neurons affected—primary lateral sclerosis (PLS) and progressive muscular atrophy (PMA), both having a better outlook than generalized ALS.[1] The identification of biomarkers upon diagnosis will also give an indication of the rate of progression the patient can expect.[10] These biomarkers are respiratory muscle strength value, esophageal pressure, twitch trans-diaphragmatic pressure, maximal static expiratory mouth pressure, and sniff-trans-diaphragmatic.[11]

The speed of progression can be predicted by a number of factors. Faster progression is linked with bulbar onset, older age at presentation/diagnosis, the short time frame from symptoms to diagnosis, the genotype, and whether cognitive impairment is already present.[1] Many ALS patients suffer from mental health issues such as depression and anxiety. However, this is thought to be linked to their poor prognosis and experience with the disease rather than a pathological origin.[8]

4.3 Epidemiology of Amyotrophic Lateral Sclerosis

Population-based studies of ALS showed 5.1% were familial ALS (FALS) and the remainder were sporadic ALS (SALS),[12] but the distinction between the two was not as clear-cut, as the same gene mutation can be attributed to both.[13] Studies show that the *C9orf72* gene is the most common ALS mutation in European patients for both FALS and SALS, while *SOD1* is most common for Asians.[14] It further shows that both Belgium and Greece have a 50% frequency of FALS with the *C9orf72* gene mutation, followed by Finland with 46.4%. Koreans have the highest frequency of *SOD1* mutations with 54.7%, followed by the Russians and Finnish with 50% and 42.9%, respectively.[14]

An overall pooled worldwide ALS crude incidence based on 44 population-based studies shows 1.75 (1.55–1.96)/100,000 person-years of follow-up (PYFU) and 1.68 (1.50–1.85)/100,000 PYFU after standardization on the U.S. population.[4]

4.3.1 Incidence

Studies conducted in the United Kingdom and the United States between multiethnicities highlight heterogeneity of incidence rates. Hispanics, African Americans, and Asian populations display lower crude incidence compared to Caucasians.[4]

4.3.2 Prevalence

In the 1990s the prevalence of SALS in western countries was an average of 5.2 (2.7–7.4)/100,000 and the lifetime risk by the age of 70 was estimated to be 1 in 400 with a male-to-female ratio of 1.5:1.[15] It was noted that prevalence of ALS is 50 to 100 times higher in parts of Japan, Guam, Kii peninsula of Japan, and Guinea than any other part of the world.[15,16]

4.3.3 Mortality

The estimated mortality rate for ALS was 1.84 (1.54–2.55)/100,000 per year in U.S. population, with the mean age of onset for SALS being between 55 and 65 years and only 5% before the age of 30 years.[15] Bulbar onset is most common in women and in older age groups, with 43% over the age of 70 years compared to 15% below the age of 30.[15] On the contrary, FALS has an onset a decade earlier than SALS and affects male and female equally, in addition to shorter survival.[15]

4.4 Etiology and Pathogenesis of Amyotrophic Lateral Sclerosis

ALS has a multifactorial pathogenesis with a cellular presentation of "cytoplasmic inclusions containing aggregated/ubiquitinated proteins as well as RNAs."[12,16] The intracellular mechanism involved in the pathogenesis includes protein misfolding with endoplasmic reticulum (ER) stress, impaired autophagy, and damage to the cytoskeleton (▶ Fig. 4.1).[12] It also presents other cellular physiology affecting and contributing to the complexities of the disease. These comprise RNA processing and mitochondrial homeostasis, increased oxidative stress, enhanced excitotoxic pathways, reduced neurotrophic support, glial inflammatory responses oriented toward a harmful side, and many of these encompassed by probable genetic predispositions (▶ Fig. 4.2).[12]

At present, ALS has unknown etiology.[17] In previous years there were very few preexisting genes or symptoms that led to an accurate

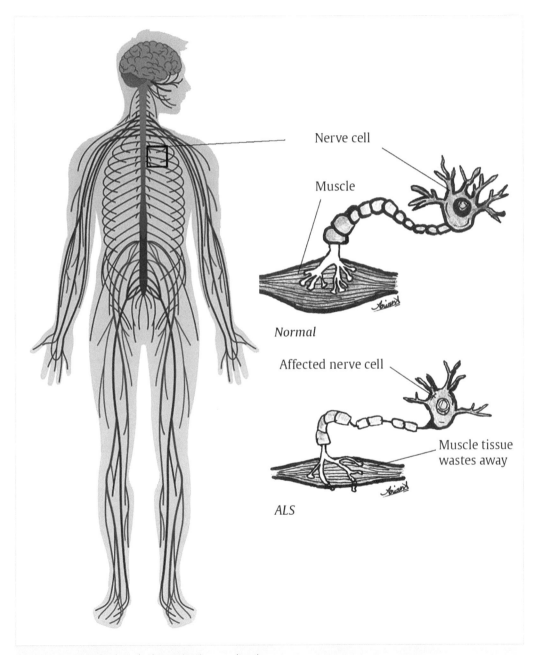

Fig. 4.1 Amyotrophic lateral sclerosis (ALS) nerve disorder.

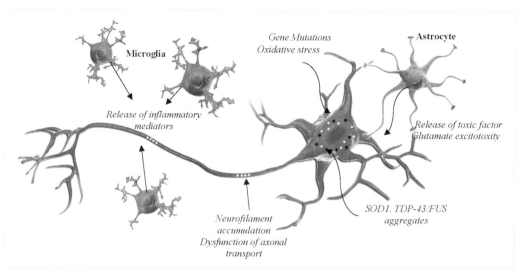

Fig. 4.2 Pathogenesis mechanisms involved in amyotrophic lateral sclerosis (ALS).

possible diagnosis.[18] These were classified as sporadic ALS (SALS), with unknown familial history, or familial ALS (FALS), a presence of ALS from first-degree or second-degree relatives.[18] Recently, there has been significant research discoveries that have led to findings of possible genetic malfunctions causing ALS.[19] Meta-analysis studies have identified *C9orf72, TARDBP, FUS,* and *SOD1,* as "The Big Four" gene mutations possibly leading to the development of ALS.[14]

4.5 Genetic Component of Amyotrophic Lateral Sclerosis

4.5.1 SOD1 (Superoxide Dismutase 1 Gene)

The *SOD1* gene was the first gene linked to some ALS cases in 1993.[20] Its native function is to catalyze the reduction of superoxide (O_2^-) with ambient protons to yield O_2 and hydrogen peroxide (H_2O_2).[21] The *SOD1* gene is an enzyme that works as an antioxidizing agent. A mutation of the *SOD1* gene no longer produces the Cu-Zn superoxide dismutase enzyme. This leads to the destruction of the mitochondria and other cellular organelles, leading to a

destruction of large groups of cells due to increased free radicals.[22] The consensus in the ALS field is that *SOD1* mutants acquire a toxic function. In other words, mutations in *SOD1* convert this otherwise helpful superoxide radical scavenging enzyme into a toxic protein that causes ALS.[20]

4.5.2 C9orf72 (Chromosome 9 Open Reading Frame 72)

The *C9orf72* (G_4C_2) gene provides instructions for making a protein that is found abundantly in neurons found in the cerebral cortex of the brain. It is likely to also play a role in RNA processing.[23] The diagnosis of *C9orf72* in relation to ALS is established by distinguishing a heterozygous pathogenic GGGGCC (G_4C_2) hexanucleotide repeat expansion on genetic molecular testing.[19] The prevalence of ALS is estimated at 4–8:100,000, with an average *C9orf72* (G_4C_2) hexanucleotide repeat expansion frequency in ALS patient cohorts of 10%.

4.5.3 TARDBP (TAR DNA-Binding Protein 43)

The *TARDBP* gene codes for DNA-binding protein 43 (TDP-43). This protein is found within the cell nucleus in most tissues and is involved in many of the steps of protein production.[24] The TDP-43 protein regulates DNA transcription. Single protein amino acid changes in the TDP-43 protein regulate most mutations. The majority of these changes affect the region of the protein involved in mRNA processing, potentially obstructing the production of other proteins.[24] These changes cause the protein to fold incorrectly, forming proteins found in nerve cells that control muscle movement in some people with ALS. It is unclear whether TDP-43 protein clumps cause the nerve cell death that leads to ALS or if they are a by-product of a dying cell. Frontal-temporal dementia has also been found to exist in patients with ALS from TDP-43 mutations.[24]

4.5.4 FUS (Fused in Sarcoma)

The *FUS* gene, similar to TARDP, is found within the cell nucleus in most tissues and is involved in many of the steps of protein production.[25] The *FUS* gene attaches itself to DNA and regulates transcription, also helping in processing mRNA. By cutting and rearranging mRNA molecules in multiple ways, the *FUS* protein regulates the production of various versions of certain proteins.[25] The mutation in the *FUS* gene may hinder the movement of mRNA out of the cell nucleus, which results in *FUS* protein and RNA being clumped together. These clumps have been found in nerve cells that control muscle movement in some people with ALS.[25]

4.6 Diagnostic Evaluation of Amyotrophic Lateral Sclerosis

4.6.1 Disease Identification

Identifying and diagnosing ALS can be challenging. To properly identify and correctly diagnose the condition, a thorough review of signs and symptoms must be performed (▶ Fig. 4.3).[9] ALS is only accurately diagnosed after symptoms worsen, and the disease has matured.[9] Due to previous lack of knowledge surrounding the origin of the disease, it has become difficult to not only cure but diagnose until very late into its progression.[1] ALS often begins simply as muscle weakness. This condition will worsen over time, eventually leading to a total loss of motor function.[9] Two main courses of progression generally occur: Limb onset individuals will begin loosing coordination while running or walking; Bulbar onset symptoms include difficulty swallowing or talking.[9] A further progression leads to a difficulty swallowing (dysphagia), speaking (dysarthria), and loss of motor control (spasticity and hyperreflexia). Another sign of ALS is the weakening of intercostal muscles of the diaphragm leading to decreased lung capacity and severe respiratory problems.[9]

A newer alternative diagnostic tool is the identification of genes that are associated with ALS.[9] *SOD1* is one such gene, which is commonly associated with FALS.[22] A possible treatment is an experimental therapeutic agent that has the potential to target the *SOD1* gene promoting intracellular copper uptake, thus promoting the function of this gene.[26] A correlation between individuals with ALS and high levels of glutamate is also a biomarker under observation.[27] A diagnosis of ALS from glutamate levels should not be inferred, nor a causation as the link is still being studied.[27]

4.6.2 Medical History

A thorough medical history should be employed when diagnosing ALS.[28] Individual medical histories seem to provide more accurate data as opposed to a family medical history. One reason may be due to only 10% of those diagnosed with ALS have family members diagnosed with the same disease.[28] A correlation, not causation, has been discovered among those with frequent drug use, pesticide exposure, and contact sports.[28] Other factors in a medical history influencing an individual personal propensity to ALS can also include exposure to heavy metals and weak magnetic fields.[29] Accurate medical histories and diagnostic tests are important, as those showing early symptoms can be treated with noninvasive treatments including positive pressure

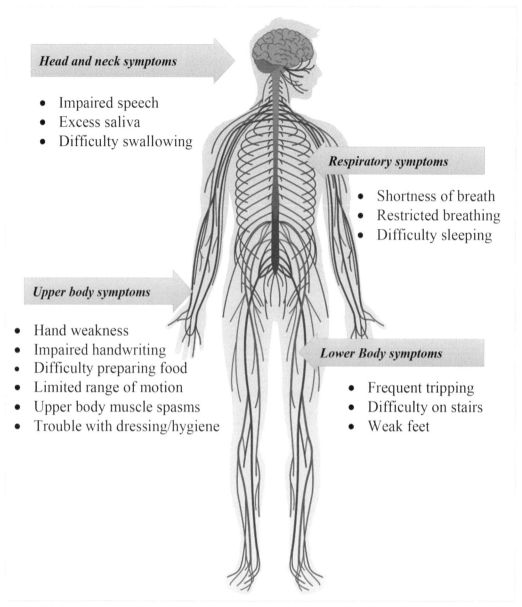

Head and neck symptoms

- Impaired speech
- Excess saliva
- Difficulty swallowing

Respiratory symptoms

- Shortness of breath
- Restricted breathing
- Difficulty sleeping

Upper body symptoms

- Hand weakness
- Impaired handwriting
- Difficulty preparing food
- Limited range of motion
- Upper body muscle spasms
- Trouble with dressing/hygiene

Lower Body symptoms

- Frequent tripping
- Difficulty on stairs
- Weak feet

Fig. 4.3 Symptoms of amyotrophic lateral sclerosis (ALS).

ventilation (NIPPV) and percutaneous gastrostomy (PEG), exhibiting higher survival rates.[30]

4.6.3 Physical Examination

A physical exam is conducted by a neurologist where questions about the patient's symptoms, family history, and medical history are explored.[31] Second, the neurologist will look for specific signs of ALS such as slurred speech, certain muscles becoming rigid and shrinking in size, twitching of muscles, and weakening of muscles on one area of the body, mouth, or tongue.[32] Slurring of speech is linked to this weakening of the muscles in the mouth and tongue[32]

4.6.4 Challenges of Implementing Physical Exams in the Clinic

The first challenge is working around the physical limitations of the ALS patient.[33] For example, the patient may have weaknesses in the upper extremity, difficulty in speech, fatigue, and/or mild depression.[32] The second challenge will be to complete the procedure with necessary structure if the patient is impulsive and distracted.[33] Third challenge is keeping in contact with the caregiver over the telephone and completing the caregiver behavioral report inventory.[33]

4.6.5 Laboratory Testing

There are currently no specific laboratory tests to diagnose ALS accurately. However, several motor neuron and muscle activity tests exist that either confirms the presence of lower motor neuron and upper motor neuron degeneration, or excludes the possibility of other disease processes.[34] Electrodiagnostic testing is performed in patients presenting motor neuron degeneration and involves peripheral nerve conduction studies (NCS) and needle electromyography (EMG).[35] Peripheral NCS evaluates motor, sensory, and F-wave nerve conduction that helps to narrow the diagnostic field for motor neurodegenerative diseases.[35] In addition, needle EMG is used to evaluate abnormal neurogenic changes, particularly with lower motor neurons, and can detect positive sharp waves, fibrillations, and fasciculation potentials that all support the diagnosis of ALS.[35] A recent study has included the use of muscle ultrasonography in combination with needle EMG to reduce patient discomfort and anxiety.[36] Furthermore, advanced magnetic resonance imaging (MRI) techniques, as well as blood and urine tests, can also be performed in order to eliminate other pathologies that may mimic the early symptoms of ALS.[37]

4.7 Medical Management and Treatment of Amyotrophic Lateral Sclerosis

4.7.1 Pharmacological Treatment

Riluzole is currently the only widely available drug used for the treatment of ALS and therapy should be initiated as soon as possible after diagnosis.[11] Riluzole is a neuroprotective drug known to inhibit the release of glutamate in the CNS and block the excitability of motor neurons.[38] Oral administration of 100 mg of riluzole daily has shown to increase the probability of surviving 1 year by 9% and prolongs median survival by 2 to 3 months.[39] The drug's role in decelerating the progression of the disease and prolonging the survival of patients with ALS is still unknown. However, there are several other therapeutic drugs currently being tested in clinical trials.[39]

Edaravone was recently approved to treat ALS patients in Japan during 2015 and in the United States during May 2017.[23] The drug is a free radical scavenger that protects the CNS against oxidative stresses, with reports suggesting that Edaravone slows the progression of functional decline; however, its effect on survival times is still uncertain.[23]

A combination of Dextromethorphan (20 mg) and Quinidine sulfate (10 mg) twice daily has shown to be efficacious in treating ALS pseudobulbar-affected patient and improving their quality of life.[34] Selective serotonin reuptake inhibitors (such as Fluvoxamine), tricyclic antidepressants, and some serotonin-norepinephrine reuptake inhibitors have also been beneficial in suppressing pseudobulbar effect.[40]

4.7.2 Respiratory Management

Respiratory failure is the leading cause of death in ALS patients, with respiratory muscle weakness giving a significant indication of the quality of life.[41] It is important to regularly discuss treatment and care plans with ALS patients before the disease progresses to a terminal phase. The timing of initiating ventilation support can be critical due to the risk of death by acute respiratory failure or ventilator dependence before sufficient planning has occurred.[41]

The management of early respiratory complications involving sleep-related symptoms (such as dyspnea and orthopnea) utilizes noninvasive positive pressure ventilation (NIPPV).[41] If tolerated, NIPPV has shown to preserve the function of oral feeding and speech, reduce the cost and dependence on caregivers, improve the overall quality of life of patients, and prolong survival by 5 to 20 months.[42]

For long-term respiratory support, invasive tracheostomy ventilation is available for patients if previous measures have not adequately maintained alveolar ventilation.[41] Although this type of treatment extends survival by an average of 5 years,[42] the patients' quality of life is not maintained. Being ventilator dependent while the disease progresses will inevitably lead to complete paralysis and loss of communication.[42] Physicians should respect patient autonomy if they refuse or withdraw from any treatment.

4.7.3 Malnutrition

Malnutrition and weight loss are predictors of survival and may occur due to dysphagia, muscle degeneration, poor appetite due to depression, and a hypermetabolic state.[41,43] ALS patients should be referred to a speech-and-language therapist who can give postural and swallowing advice to avoid choking and aspiration.[42] Dysphagia can be managed with changes in food and fluid consistency and parental feeding.[41] Percutaneous endoscopic gastrostomy (PEG) is prescribed for long-term maintenance of nutrition as treatment is well-tolerated by ALS patients and shows improvements to the quality of life.[11]

4.7.4 Pain Management

Quality of life is greatly impacted by pain and muscle cramps experienced daily by ALS patients. The use of nonsteroidal anti-inflammatory drugs, nonopioid analgesics, opioids, muscle relaxants, botulinum toxin, and physical therapy are some of the ways that pain, cramps, and spasms can be managed.[44]

4.7.5 Fatigue

Fatigue is reported in 83% of ALS patients and is shown to be a multifactorial manifestation linked with depression, dyspnea, and sleepiness.[45,46] Studies have found that 200 or 400 mg/day of modafinil for 2 weeks reduces the symptoms of fatigue; however, side effects include diarrhea, headaches, nervousness, and insomnia.[47]

4.7.6 Palliative Care

There are currently no curative treatments for ALS, so the primary focus in managing the disease heavily involves palliative care and alleviating the symptoms that may develop throughout the course of the disease.[42] Improving the quality of life of patients and their families is the main goal of palliative care.[42] It is important to discuss end-of-life issues with the patient and their families, with advanced treatment planning (including options for respiratory ventilation and enteric feeding) occurring soon after diagnosis.[40]

Receiving specialized care at a multidisciplinary ALS clinic also enables patients to reach maximal function, independence, and overall quality of life as the disease progresses.[42] Taking this holistic approach to manage the disease also shows a better prognosis as median survival of these patients is extended by 3 to 7 months when compared to those being treated at a general neurology clinic.[48]

Patients' autonomy should always be respected by family members and any physician or specialist treating the patient. In the final stages of the disease, hospice services are crucial in facilitating a peaceful and dignified death.[40]

4.8 Management of Dental Patients with Amyotrophic Lateral Sclerosis

4.8.1 Sialorrhea

Sialorrhea in ALS patients can be treated with anticholinergic medication. The type of drug and dosage is determined by the severity and frequency of drooling.[40] Side effects of these drugs include constipation, urinary retention, orthostatic hypotension, and fatigue. It is recommended to initiate the use of a stool softener when commencing anticholinergic therapy.[40]

Botulinum toxin injections to the submandibular or parotid glands have also shown success in treating sialorrhea in patients who are resistant to conventional medical therapy.[40] Beta-blockers such as Propranolol (10 mg) or Metoprolol (50 mg) twice daily can be combined with anticholinergics to reduce viscosity and aid expectoration of mucus formed due to bronchial secretions.[42]

4.8.2 Dental Modifications

ALS manifestations can affect the dental care of ALS patients.[49] Since there is a high incidence of dysphagia in ALS individuals, it is often necessary to modify dental treatment.[50] First, the dental operator may need to modify the positioning of the patient.[51] Saliva may pool in the oral cavity, and the limited mobility associated with lack of coordination of muscles can create difficulties in protecting the airway.[52] Thus, a semisupine position is suggested to improve patient comfort because this position makes aspirating excess saliva an easier task.[52] Second, it is important to have more than one dental assistant to prevent saliva from pooling and interfering with the dental treatment.[49] Third, short appointments or appointments with breaks in between the treatment may enhance patient-comfort.[50] This is because ALS patients experience spasticity and muscle weakness that makes it difficult to keep the mouth open for the duration of a regular appointment.[50] In addition, using a bite block might be helpful in keeping the mouth open during the dental treatment.[49]

Lastly, the gagging tendency can be reduced by using a pea-sized amount of gel toothpaste without an extra fresh or mint label on it.[52]

Using local anesthetic (LA) is ideal to combat the gagging problem seen in ALS patients.[52] LA also allows the completion of complicated treatments in one session.[52] However, the disadvantage of using LA or muscle relaxants in ALS patients is that it can lead to prolonged neuromuscular paralysis and postoperative ventilation.[50] Since conventional volatile anesthetics have unpredictable half-lives and wake-up times, research suggests the use of total intravenous anesthesia (TIVA) without using muscle relaxants.[52]

4.8.3 Difficulties with Personal Oral Hygiene

Changes in the function of patient's hands or arms may cause difficulties in holding a toothbrush, squeezing toothpaste from a tube, flossing in between teeth, opening the lid of a mouth-rinse bottle, or putting dentures in and out from the oral cavity.[51] In addition, changes in the function of the tongue may cause difficulties in clearing food from the mouth, spitting after brushing, rinsing the mouth, and closing the mouth, making it difficult to keep the oral cavity moist.[49]

4.8.4 Risks Associated with Lack of Proper Oral Hygiene

If the patient is constantly breathing from the mouth, there is an increased chance of having halitosis due to dry mouth.[49] In addition, there is a high chance of developing gum disease, dental caries, dental abscesses, cellulitis, and mouth sores, which are all commonly seen dental diseases in ALS patients.[51] There is also an increased risk of developing pneumonia (lung infection) by aspiration of bacteria from the oral cavity.[52]

4.8.5 Improving Oral Hygiene in ALS Patients

Home care oral hygiene practices may need to be modified due to a loss in the function of muscles.[49] Toothpaste dispensers (hands-free or pumps), electrical toothbrushes, and floss holders can be used by those patients without a caretaker.[51] If flossing is still difficult with the use of a floss holder, an alternative to flossing is using an oral irrigator.[51] The dentist can introduce a different brushing technique to make brushing easier for the patient.[49] Those patients who have severe spasticity and loss of motor function will need to bring a family member or a care provider to the dental appointment to take note on the nutrition plan and home care oral hygiene procedures for the patient.[50]

The caretaker should brush the patient's teeth twice a day using a soft-bristled toothbrush and fluoride toothpaste to prevent bacteria and plaque build-up.[51] This is especially important before bed to prevent bacteria from entering the upper airway during sleep.[51] All ALS patients should obtain more frequent dental visits to keep the oral health in check.[50]

Food intake for ALS patients can be affected by swallowing difficulties.[51] Therefore, the dentist may refer the patient to the nutritionist for nutritional counseling. Educating the patient on oral health is important because it helps the patient understand how nutrition impacts oral tissues.[51] By discussing this with the ALS patient, the dentist and the patient can derive an individualized nutrition plan that will help the current physiological needs of the patient.[51]

4.9 Coordination of Care between Dentist and Physician

Medicine and dentistry interlink at many levels. At the outset of the 1900s, the focal infection theory suggested that systemic manifestations could be traced to dental infections. With the emergence of antibiotic therapy, this medical–dental relationship was largely separated until recently.[53] The link between periodontal diseases and heart ailments among other findings has reestablished some interest in the role of oral health and general health.[53] In accordance with recent research outcomes, the reemerging collaboration of the physician and dentist is essential for the well-being of people across a broad spectrum of systemic conditions.[54]

Interprofessional collaboration is a means to achieve greater resource efficiency, standards of care, the continuity of care by minimizing duplication and negating the gaps in service. An obstacle pervading the unity of the medical–dental relationship has its foundations in the educational model.[55] Medical doctors and dentists are trained as distinct professionals that exhibit separate responsibilities. Dentists are trained to focus on the diagnosis and treatment of oral diseases, devoting much of their skill to restoration and replacement techniques, although the need for this intervention has declined.[55] On the contrary, doctors are trained to complement overall health without training in oral health problems.[54] Medical and dental students should be given the opportunity to integrate as part of their educational development. This is currently implemented in some European and U.S. medical schools, with the onset of oral health curricula as part of the medical undergraduate training.[56] Some dental schools are expanding their curricula to advocate an "oral physician" model, with the understanding of systemic disease pathophysiology and the importance of homogenizing the dental–medical relationship for a greater health outcome.[55]

As mentioned earlier, a multidisciplinary clinical coordination should be a high priority for managing patients with ALS to optimize the healthcare delivery, increase the survival rate, and improve the quality of life of the patient.[57] In an evidence-based recommendation study, general principles of ALS management had been established to guide clinicians in managing patients with the disease.[57] The patient survival and coordination of care were also examined, resulting in fewer hospitalizations and increased use of Riluzole, PEG, and NIV. The mean survival of the patient was longer, received more aids and appliances, and had a higher quality of life. Therefore, a multidisciplinary clinic that includes a medical doctor, physical therapist, occupational therapist, speech pathologist, dietician, social worker, respiratory therapist, and nurse has been recommended as a more efficient method for the delivery of care.[57]

Effective management of symptoms is, at present, a primary goal of ALS patient care.[57] Furthermore, the dedicated monitoring by a dentist would be essential to achieve this objective.[58] Oral conditions such as glossitis, periodontal diseases, caries, stomatitis, and halitosis frequently remain undiagnosed due to the inability of the patient to communicate discomfort and pain.[58] A dentist's role in managing the oral health in conjunction with a multidisciplinary collaboration is fundamental to enhance patient quality of life and prevent the further onset of systemic complications that could risk a further physical imbalance.[57,58]

Invasive or oral surgical dental interventions of a patient presenting with ALS should preferably be planned in conjunction with a medical team, and in some cases, the neurologist.[59] In addition, dental care should be coordinated with the physician to assess critical conditions of ALS patients, especially those with bulbar onset. Despite receiving close medical attention, patients with bulbar onset quite commonly neglect oral health, further declining in overall health.[58]

ALS is a progressive neurodegenerative disease that has significant effects on functionality, independency, and overall quality of life. ALS has an unknown etiology which leads to a challenging diagnostic process that can delay the commencement of management of the disease. Symptomatic alleviation is utilized for ALS as there are currently no curative treatments available; however, several therapeutic drugs are currently being tested in clinical trials. Modifications to dental treatment are required to ensure the comfort and protection of ALS patients. In addition, home care oral hygiene practices should be modified progressively for patients with ALS, and dentist visits should occur more frequently due to a higher risk of developing oral diseases. Therefore, multidisciplinary clinical coordination is essential for optimizing health care delivery, increasing survival rate, and enhancing the quality of life of ALS patients.

References

[1] Al-Chalabi A, Hardiman O. The epidemiology of ALS: a conspiracy of genes, environment and time. Nat Rev Neurol. 2013; 9(11):617–628

[2] Brites D, Vaz AR. Microglia centered pathogenesis in ALS: insights in cell interconnectivity. Front Cell Neurosci. 2014; 8:117

[3] Gerber YN, Sabourin JC, Rabano M, Vivanco Md, Perrin FE. Early functional deficit and microglial disturbances in a mouse model of amyotrophic lateral sclerosis. PLoS One. 2012; 7(4):e36000

[4] Luna J, Logroscino G, Couratier P, Marin B. Current issues in ALS epidemiology: variation of ALS occurrence between populations and physical activity as a risk factor. Rev Neurol (Paris). 2017; 173(5):244–253

[5] Mehta P, Antao V, Kaye W, et al. Prevalence of amyotrophic lateral sclerosis: United States, 2010–2011. MMWR. 2014; 25 (7):1–14

[6] Turner MR, Bowser R, Bruijn L, et al. Mechanisms, models and biomarkers in amyotrophic lateral sclerosis. Amyotroph Lateral Scler Frontotemporal Degener. 2013; 14 Suppl 1:19–32

[7] Goldstein LH, Abrahams S. Changes in cognition and behaviour in amyotrophic lateral sclerosis: nature of impairment and implications for assessment. Lancet Neurol. 2013; 12(4): 368–380

[8] Hogden A, Foley G, Henderson RD, James N, Aoun SM. Amyotrophic lateral sclerosis: improving care with a multidisciplinary approach. J Multidiscip Healthc. 2017; 10:205–215

[9] Bede P, Iyer PM, Finegan E, Omer T, Hardiman O. Virtual brain biopsies in amyotrophic lateral sclerosis: diagnostic classification based on in vivo pathological patterns. Neuroimage Clin. 2017; 15:653–658

[10] Gaiani A, Martinelli I, Bello L, et al. Diagnostic and prognostic biomarkers in amyotrophic lateral sclerosis: neurofilament light chain levels in definite subtypes of disease. JAMA Neurol. 2017; 74(5):525–532

[11] Mathis S, Couratier P, Julian A, Vallat J-M, Corcia P, Le Masson G. Management and therapeutic perspectives in amyotrophic lateral sclerosis. Expert Rev Neurother. 2017; 17(3):263–276

[12] Geloso MC, Corvino V, Marchese E, Serrano A, Michetti F, D'Ambrosi N. The dual role of microglia in ALS: mechanisms and therapeutic approaches. Front Aging Neurosci. 2017; 9: 242

[13] Turner MR, Al-Chalabi A, Chio A, et al. Genetic Screening in Sporadic ALS and FTD. BMJ Publishing Group Ltd; 2017

[14] Veldink JH. ALS Genetic Epidemiology: How Simplex is the Genetic Epidemiology of ALS? BMJ Publishing Group Ltd; 2017

[15] Wijesekera LC, Leigh PN. Amyotrophic lateral sclerosis. Orphanet J Rare Dis. 2009; 4(1):3

[16] Bonafede R, Mariotti R. ALS pathogenesis and therapeutic approaches: the role of mesenchymal stem cells and extracellular vesicles. Front Cell Neurosci. 2017; 11:80

[17] Logroscino G, Traynor BJ, Hardiman O, et al. EURALS. Descriptive epidemiology of amyotrophic lateral sclerosis: new evidence and unsolved issues. J Neurol Neurosurg Psychiatry. 2008; 79(1):6–11

[18] Byrne S, Walsh C, Lynch C, et al. Rate of familial amyotrophic lateral sclerosis: a systematic review and meta-analysis. J Neurol Neurosurg Psychiatry. 2011; 82(6):623–627

[19] Cruts M, Engelborghs S, van der Zee J, Van Broeckhoven C. C9orf72-Related Amyotrophic Lateral Sclerosis and Frontotemporal Dementia. GeneReviews; 2015

[20] DA B. Nature News [Internet]. Nature Publishing Group; 2017 [cited August 28, 2017]. Available at: https://www.nature.com/scitable/topicpage/the-role-of-sod1-in-amyotrophic-lateral-131764166. Accessed May 16, 2019

[21] Minikel. How do SOD1 mutations cause ALS? 2015 [cited August 28, 2017]. Available at: http://www.cureffi.org/2015/04/30/how-do-sod1-mutations-cause-als. Accessed May 16, 2019

[22] Kumar V, Rahman S, Choudhry H, et al. Computing disease-linked SOD1 mutations: deciphering protein stability and patient-phenotype relations. Sci Rep. 2017; 7(1):4678

[23] Mullard A. FDA approves first new ALS drug in over 20 years. Nat Rev Drug Discov. 2017; 16(6):375

[24] Liu X, Yang L, Tang L, Chen L, Liu X, Fan D. DCTN1 gene analysis in Chinese patients with sporadic amyotrophic lateral sclerosis. PLoS One. 2017; 12(8):e0182572

[25] Zhou T, Ahmad TK, Gozda K, Truong J, Kong J, Namaka M. Implications of white matter damage in amyotrophic lateral sclerosis (Review). Mol Med Rep. 2017; 16(4):4379–4392

[26] Tokuda E, Furukawa Y. Copper homeostasis as a therapeutic target in amyotrophic lateral sclerosis with SOD1 mutations. Int J Mol Sci. 2016; 17(5):636

[27] Bonifacino T, Cattaneo L, Gallia E, et al. In-vivo effects of knocking-down metabotropic glutamate receptor 5 in the SOD1G93A mouse model of amyotrophic lateral sclerosis. Neuropharmacology. 2017; 123:433–445

[28] Feddermann-Demont N, Junge A, Weber KP, Weller M, Dvořák J, Tarnutzer AA. Prevalence of potential sports-associated risk factors in Swiss amyotrophic lateral sclerosis patients. Brain Behav. 2017; 7(4):e00630

[29] Koeman T, Slottje P, Schouten LJ, et al. Occupational exposure and amyotrophic lateral sclerosis in a prospective cohort. Occup Environ Med. 2017; 74(8):578–585

[30] Lavernhe S, Antoine J-C, Court-Fortune I, et al. Home care organization impacts patient management and survival in ALS. Amyotroph Lateral Scler Frontotemporal Degener. 2017; 18(7–8):562–568

[31] Hillel A, Dray T, Miller R, et al. Presentation of ALS to the otolaryngologist/head and neck surgeon: getting to the neurologist. Neurology. 1999; 53(8) Suppl 5:S22–S25, discussion S35–S36

[32] Kinsley L, Siddique T. Amyotrophic Lateral Sclerosis Overview. In: Pagon RA, Adam MP, Ardinger HH, Wallace SE, Amemiya A, Bean LJH, et al, eds. GeneReviews(R). Seattle, WA: 1993

[33] Achi EY, Rudnicki SA. ALS and frontotemporal dysfunction: a review. Neurol Res Int. 2012; 2012:806306

[34] Brooks BR, Thisted RA, Appel SH, et al. AVP-923 ALS Study Group. Treatment of pseudobulbar affect in ALS with dextromethorphan/quinidine: a randomized trial. Neurology. 2004; 63(8):1364–1370

[35] Joyce NC, Carter GT. Electrodiagnosis in persons with amyotrophic lateral sclerosis. PM R. 2013; 5(5) Suppl:S89–S95

[36] Grimm A, Prell T, Décard BF, et al. Muscle ultrasonography as an additional diagnostic tool for the diagnosis of amyotrophic lateral sclerosis. Clin Neurophysiol. 2015; 126(4):820–827

[37] Wang S, Melhem ER, Poptani H, Woo JH. Neuroimaging in amyotrophic lateral sclerosis. Neurotherapeutics. 2011; 8(1):63–71

[38] Miller RG, Mitchell JD, Lyon M, Moore DH. Riluzole for amyotrophic lateral sclerosis (ALS)/motor neuron disease (MND). Cochrane Database Syst Rev. 2007; 1(1):CD001447

[39] Martinez A, Palomo Ruiz MD, Perez DI, Gil C. Drugs in clinical development for the treatment of amyotrophic lateral sclerosis. Expert Opin Investig Drugs. 2017; 26(4):403–414

[40] Jackson CE, McVey AL, Rudnicki S, Dimachkie MM, Barohn RJ. Symptom management and end-of-life care in amyotrophic lateral sclerosis. Neurol Clin. 2015; 33(4):889–908

[41] Phukan J, Hardiman O. The management of amyotrophic lateral sclerosis. J Neurol. 2009; 256(2):176–186

[42] Thibodeaux LS, Gutierrez A. Management of symptoms in amyotrophic lateral sclerosis. Curr Treat Options Neurol. 2008; 10(2):77–85

[43] Stambler N, Charatan M, Cedarbaum JM, ALS CNTF Treatment Study Group. Prognostic indicators of survival in ALS. Neurology. 1998; 50(1):66–72

[44] Pizzimenti A, Aragona M, Onesti E, Inghilleri M. Depression, pain and quality of life in patients with amyotrophic lateral sclerosis: a cross-sectional study. Funct Neurol. 2013; 28(2):115–119

[45] Ramirez C, Piemonte ME, Callegaro D, Da Silva HC. Fatigue in amyotrophic lateral sclerosis: frequency and associated factors. Amyotroph Lateral Scler. 2008; 9(2):75–80

[46] Nicholson K, Murphy A, McDonnell E, et al. Improving symptom management for people with amyotrophic lateral sclerosis. Muscle Nerve.

[47] Carter GT, Weiss MD, Lou JS, et al. Modafinil to treat fatigue in amyotrophic lateral sclerosis: an open label pilot study. Am J Hosp Palliat Care. 2005; 22(1):55–59

[48] Traynor BJ, Alexander M, Corr B, Frost E, Hardiman O. Effect of a multidisciplinary amyotrophic lateral sclerosis (ALS) clinic on ALS survival: a population based study, 1996–2000. J Neurol Neurosurg Psychiatry. 2003; 74(9):1258–1261

[49] Parsons KM, Schneider AJ. Clinical considerations for treating the dental patient with ALS. RDH 2014. Available at: https://www.rdhmag.com/home/article/16404134/clinical-considerations-for-treating-the-dental-patient-with-als. Accessed May 16, 2019

[50] Andersen PM, Borasio GD, Dengler R, et al. EALSC Working Group. Good practice in the management of amyotrophic lateral sclerosis: clinical guidelines. An evidence-based review with good practice points. Amyotroph Lateral Scler. 2007; 8(4):195–213

[51] KH K. Oral care for people living with ALS: The ALS Association. 2014 Available at: http://www.alsa.org/als-care/resources/publications. Accessed May 16, 2019

[52] Austin S, Kumar S, Russell D, da Silva E, Boote M. Dental treatment for a patient with motor neurone disease completed under total intravenous anaesthesia: a case report. J Disability Oral Health. 2011; 12(3):124

[53] Casamassimo PS. Relationships between oral and systemic health. Pediatr Clin North Am. 2000; 47(5):1149–1157

[54] Zhang S, Lo EC, Chu C-H. Attitude and awareness of medical and dental students towards collaboration between medical and dental practice in Hong Kong. BMC Oral Health. 2015; 15(1):53

[55] Hendricson WD, Cohen PA. Oral health care in the 21st century: implications for dental and medical education. Acad Med. 2001; 76(12):1181–1206

[56] Migliorati CA, Madrid C. The interface between oral and systemic health: the need for more collaboration. Clin Microbiol Infect. 2007; 13 Suppl 4:11–16

[57] Miller RG, Jackson CE, Kasarskis EJ, et al. Quality Standards Subcommittee of the American Academy of Neurology. Practice parameter update: the care of the patient with amyotrophic lateral sclerosis: drug, nutritional, and respiratory therapies (an evidence-based review): report of the Quality Standards Subcommittee of the American Academy of Neurology. Neurology. 2009; 73(15):1218–1226

[58] Erriu M, Pili FMG, Denotti G, Garau V. Black hairy tongue in a patient with amyotrophic lateral sclerosis. J Int Soc Prev Community Dent. 2016; 6(1):80–83

[59] Patton LL. The ADA Practical Guide to Patients with Medical Conditions: John Wiley & Sons; 2015

5 Alzheimer Disease

Haleh Vosgha

Abstract

Alzheimer disease with progressive impairment of memory and other cognitive functions is the common cause of dementia. It is an increasingly prevalent condition in an aging population with many oral- and dental-related implications. Primarily with a decline in mental status, Alzheimer disease presents with no motor, sensory, or coordination problems in the early stages. Dementia is a set of behavioral and psychological symptoms associated with the loss of memory, language, and recognition in various stages of the disease that reduce the ability to perform everyday activities. The patient's stage of Alzheimer disease will be the determinant for the practitioner as to which precautions and procedures they will undertake in the best interest of the patient. Treatment options available for the condition have shown clinical success in terms of symptom improvement and cognitive function; however, they are not devoid of adverse effects. Collaboration with other health professionals is imperative for awareness of drug interactions, formulation of treatment plans, and improvement in the overall well-being of the patient.

Keywords: Alzheimer disease, epidemiology, pathogenesis, oral manifestations, medical management, treatment

5.1 Background of Alzheimer Disease

Alzheimer disease is the common cause of dementia, with its insidious onset causing the progressive impairment of memory and other cognitive functions. Alzheimer diagnosis relies primarily on the mental decline, with no motor, sensory, or coordination problems evident in the early stages. Currently, neuroimaging with magnetic resonance imaging and computed tomography (CT) is able to confirm the absence of other possible causes. Today there is focus on biomarkers, easily detectable by molecular imaging, such as the PET scan. It is important to understand the disease so sufferers requiring dental treatment can be catered for effectively and efficiently.

Alzheimer disease (AD) is a progressive, degenerative brain disease, and is the most common form of dementia globally. It affects up to 70% of people that suffer from dementia, with an estimated 115.4 million people predicted as sufferers by the year 2050.[1] Its incidence and prevalence is linked to the increase in age,[2] with approximately 5% of sufferers developing symptoms before the age of 65, associated with early-onset Alzheimer disease (EOAD). Of those, 85 to 90% of sufferers present with sporadic Alzheimer disease, beginning at 50+ years of age, with mainly temporal profile, similar to that of late-onset Alzheimer disease (LOAD).[2] LOAD occurs in people aged 65 and older. According to Toyota et al,[3] few differences exist behaviorally and psychologically between EOAD and LOAD, with no cognitive or dementia severity differences being displayed. The remainder 10 to 15% will have the genetic form (aggressive in nature, starting at 40 years of age).[4] Dementia is not a disease by itself, but rather a set of behavioral and psychological symptoms that are associated with specific diseases.[5] The term dementia is generally used to describe the loss of memory, language and recognition in various stages of the disease, to such an extent that it interferes with daily life.[6] According to Reisberg,[7] there are seven stages of Alzheimer disease, which include preclinical (stage 1), mild dementia (stages 2 and 3), moderate dementia (stages 4 and 5), severe dementia (stage 6), and very severe dementia (stage 7). The patient's stage of Alzheimer disease will be the determinant for the dental practitioner as to which precautions and procedures they will undertake in the best interest of the patient. This chapter will look at the background, description, epidemiology, pathogenesis/etiology, genetic components, identification, medical history, physical exams and lab testing, dental treatment of patients with the disease, and oral medicines available with regard to AD.

Early detection of AD is instrumental in slowing down the process and providing the necessary care.[8] In addition, it provides the best response to treatments and quality of life when dealing with Huntington, Parkinson, and Pick that cause irreversible dementia. Early detection enables a person to function "normally" for longer periods of time, and in some cases, reversible symptoms that mimic dementia can be identified and handled effectively. Alzheimer disease damages the human brain affecting memory, thinking, and behavior. Statistics reveal that globally, approximately 33% of people over the age of 85 have some form of dementia (LOAD).[9] However, sporadic Alzheimer disease can affect anyone of any age,[10] and familial Alzheimer disease, a rare genetic condition, usually affects people under the age of 65 (EOAD).[10]

AD was first recorded by Dr. Alois Alzheimer in 1907 when he began studying Auguste Deter, a female patient in her 50 s. Her symptoms of dementia were associated with changes taking place in her brain.[11] Until the 1970s, Alzheimer disease was considered rare; however, it was Dr. Robert Katzman who realized that senile dementia and Alzheimer disease were the same thing, with both displaying symptoms not part of the normal aging process.[12] He hypothesized that two types of AD existed: sporadic (occurring in people 65 years and older), and familial, a genetic condition affecting people in their 40 s and 50 s, both causing irreversible damage to the brain.

5.2 Description of Alzheimer Disease

The brain, with its complex network of arteries and veins and capillaries that feed the brain its required blood and oxygen needed to survive, is the most complex part of the body to treat medically.[13] As a result, the brain's blood network is separated from the rest of the body, with its intricate blood barrier protecting it from infection. If an infection does infiltrate this barrier, treatment is difficult as the molecules in antibiotics are too large to penetrate the brain's barrier. Any agent that could possibly treat Alzheimer disease needs to consist of small molecular structures able to target the brain.[14] In addition, the brain is comprised of many parts, such as the temporal lobes responsible for speech, working memory, and "higher emotions" such as empathy, morality, and regret.[15] The limbic system of the brain processes our desires and emotions,[12] while the cerebellum stores our muscle memory responsible for involuntary muscle actions, such as walking, lifting, etc.[16] The midbrain controls the heart rate and digestion and is the link between the spinal cord and the remainder of the brain. All tasks are carried out by sensitive connections via the brain's neurons, called synapses. In an average adult human brain, 100 billion neurons exist, each connected to its neighbors by 5,000 to 10,000 synapses.[17] Every second of our lives we make new connections, we learn new things, and it is in these changing connections that memories are stored, habits are formed, and personalities developed in a unique fashion as no two brains are the same.

Brain cells (neurons) communicate via the process of synapses, where signals move in chemical form across the synapse, called neurotransmitters. These pass from one neuron to the receiving neuron, which collects it using a receptor. The receiving neuron then, in turn, sends out a burst of neurotransmitters to various other brain neurons, and so the message gets relayed.[18] What Dr. Alzheimer discovered with Auguste Deter was that the outer layer of the brain, known as the cortex, had visibly undergone a permanent shrinking process caused by dying brain cells. As this part of the brain became affected, so too did Ms. Deter's ability to remember, to communicate, and to judge. Two types of plaque were also discovered in her brain, plaque outside the brain neurons, and the other inside the brain neurons, which are called "neurofibrillary tangles" (NFTs).[19] These plaque deposits hinder synapses, and the NFTs starve the neurons of food and energy. By using the technique of magnetic resonance imaging (MRI), shrinking of the brain can be detected even in the early stages of AD.[20] Alzheimer disease is progressive, initially affecting the outer portion of the brain, leading to a loss of short-term memory, and eventually long-term memory loss and other behavioral patterns become disturbed (▶ Fig. 5.1).[21]

Not a great deal is known about Alzheimer disease, or what triggers the plaque and tangle formations, in addition to the other chemical changes that occur within the brain, as this disease causes irreparable damage. To date only suspected causes have been investigated, such as environment, biochemical disturbances, and the process of the body's immune system. In the final stages of AD, the three main causes of death are pneumonia, dehydration, and malnutrition.[12] The average time frame living with Alzheimer disease is 7 to 10 years.[22] However, temporary improvement with regard to cognitive functioning, for those with mild-to-moderate Alzheimer disease, can be achieved by taking cholinergic drugs.[23] However, early detection is important to relieve the anxiety of the unknown, allowing adequate time to develop an advanced care plan. The quality of life can be maximized, and with early treatment, there is a greater chance of a favorable response to treatment, thereby prolonging progressive symptoms, resulting in lower costs overall. A new cost-effective method for early preventative detection is now being trialed, with a noninvasive eye scan that can detect signs on the retina of the eye, which has a central nervous system similar to

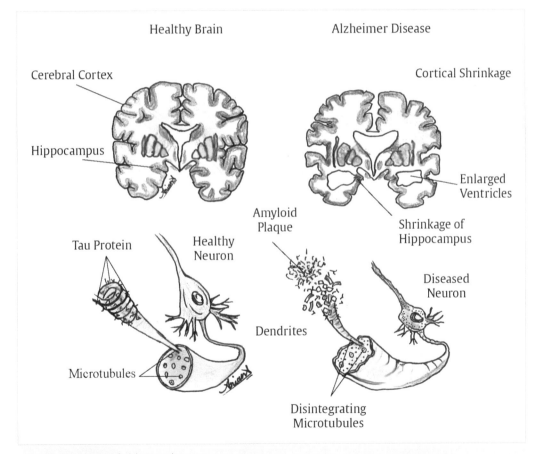

Fig. 5.1 Progression of Alzheimer disease.

that of the brain.[24] Early detection involves education about the symptoms and testing for those with a family history of Alzheimer disease.[5] The three main risk factors include a family history,[5] the apolipoprotein E4 (ApoE4) allele,[25] and age.[26] Currently, there are drugs that aim to prevent the formation of the beta-amyloid plaques by inhibiting the beta and gamma secretase. If beta-amyloid is not formed on the amyloid precursor protein (APP), it averts impairment of the synaptic function by neurodegeneration, limiting the progression of Alzheimer disease. This medication is not ideal, in that it also brings about cleavage of other proteins.[27] Nontherapeutic interventions are proving effective, with cognitive therapy being able to minimize psychological symptoms of the disease.[28]

With the age increase of the global population and consequently rise in the prevalence of Alzheimer disease, dental treatment of such patients seems more important for reduction of its associated co-morbidities.[29] Research has shown the link between periodontal disease and the progression of the neurological dysfunction in AD patients. This requires monitoring and treatment of the condition.[30,31] As a dental professional, an initial dental plan is imperative with all AD patients so that all their present and future needs can be catered for, such as written consent by the patient in the early stages of AD, the use of saliva sprays to replace patient saliva, the use of dentures to prevent further dental issue, and the use of anesthesia during some procedures. By doing this, the dental practitioner can operate in a safe environment, ensuring the best outcome for their patient.

5.3 Epidemiology of Alzheimer Disease

As human life expectancy increases so does the prevalence of Alzheimer disease (AD) among our ever-aging population. In 2016, it was estimated that 5.4 million people in America alone suffered from the disease and was most prevalent in individuals 65 years and older (5.4 million people) as opposed to

individuals 64 years and younger (200,000 people).[32] Of those individuals 65 years and older suffering from AD, it was found that 63% were female and 37% were male, showing an obvious trend between sexes.[32]

This data is found to be consistent with some of the three main risk factors reported for AD: age, a family history of AD, and the ApoE4 allele.[32] Age is one of the greatest risk factors for AD, with numerous studies around the world showing a dramatic increase in the expression of the disease over the age of 65.[32] The second risk factor, a family history of AD, has been proven by many studies to increase the likelihood of developing the disease. Whether the family history is related to the genetic presence of the ApoE4 protein or not is still currently being researched.[33] Finally, a study conducted in 2014 found that the female carriers of the ApoE4 allele more frequently went on to suffer from AD. This can be supported by data generated from a study of the prevalence of AD in Europe (2013), which showed the prevalence of AD in women was nearly double than that in men (7.13 and 3.31%).[34] Another identified risk factor for the development of AD is a periodontal disease. A retrospective cohort study was performed using the NHIRD (National Health Insurance Research Database) of Taiwan, which looked at the association between chronic periodontitis (CP) and the risk of AD, and it was concluded that patients who had CP for at least 10 years were 1.7 times more likely to develop AD than in patients who did not have CP.[35]

The 1984 guidelines and criteria published by National Institute on Aging and the Alzheimer's Association has been the standard for diagnosing AD in America until it was reviewed in 2011.[32] Traditionally, a person was diagnosed with the AD as soon as they expressed certain physical symptoms, until more recently it was suggested that the disease could be expressed even before the emergence of its symptoms,[32] which is a concept now widely accepted by most researchers.[36] If this indeed was the case, the inconsistency between definitions and diagnostic guidelines for AD makes it difficult to generate a precise figure of morbidity rates within a population, and it is thought that if there were a reliable mechanism to detect pre-symptomatic AD, there would be a much higher prevalence and incidence rates of the disease than currently reported.[32]

5.4 Pathogenesis and Etiology of Alzheimer Disease

AD was first pathologically characterized by extracellular amyloid plaques and intracellular NFTs,[37] resulting in impaired cognition characterized by memory loss, disorientation, lack of comprehension, reduced judgment, and more.[38] Despite significant evidence to support the correlation between AD and plaques and NFTs, some histopathology studies have clinically diagnosed nondemented individuals with AD.[37] A study on the molecular pathogenesis of AD in 2016 concluded that no single proposed theory can entirely clarify the pathogenesis of AD.[38] Two proposed theories on the pathophysiology of AD are the cholinergic and amyloid hypotheses.[38] Despite the fact that the mechanism of AD initiation and progression remains unclear,[39] apolipoprotein E (ApoE) has demonstrated a significant role in the pathogenesis of AD.[40]

The earliest and most severe atrophy of the brain in AD patients is in the medial temporal lobe.[41] Characteristic findings in autopsy reveal neuritic plaques (senile) and NFTs.[41] Adjunct to typical plaques and NFTs, studies have revealed a significant imbalance between reactive oxygen species (ROS) and antioxidants in AD, resulting in neural cell damage.[38] Though causation of elevated levels of ROS remains unclear, the amyloid hypothesis states that abnormal amyloid β accumulation results in the release of ROS, and released ROS may reversibly stimulate amyloid β production—resulting in a repetitive cycle that may be linked to the progression of Alzheimer disease.[38] Abnormal amyloid β polymerization and production leads to amyloid angiopathy within cerebral arteries, linked to reduced cognition and seizures in AD patients.[41]

A study on memory impairment caused by extracellular amyloid β and tau protein (T protein: a proteins that stabilizes microtubules) has demonstrated that both proteins are dependent on the expression of APP, revealing a promising therapeutic target against AD.[42] NFTs contain abnormally phosphorylated tau protein: an oligomer protein required to support axonal transport of organelles and neurotransmitters and stabilize microtubules.[41] Protein phosphatase 2A (PP2A) acts to dephosphorylate tau protein; however, genetic abnormalities in PP2A lead to the abnormal phosphorylation of tau protein, compromising function and contributing to AD pathogenesis.[43] Postmortem AD patients expressing at least one ApoE4 allele have demonstrated elevated tau phosphorylation.[43] A study on the down-regulation of PP2A has linked abnormalities in PP2A to ApoE4, stating that ApoE4 allele inheritance is the most important genetic risk factor for AD.[43] The ApoE4 allele binds to the PPP2RSE promoter region on DNA and consequently reduces PP2A activity by reducing its gene expression.[43] Abnormal changes in tau and amyloid β protein in the CNS are responsible for neuronal dysfunction in the pathogenesis of Alzheimer disease.[38]

The cholinergic hypothesis of the pathogenesis of AD suggests that cognitive impairment is attributed to cholinergic dysfunction.[44] AD is biochemically associated with a reduction in the neurotransmitter acetylcholine, choline acetyltransferase (CAT enzyme), and reduced expression of nicotinic and muscarinic receptors.[41] Nonselective muscarinic antagonists have shown to induce cognitive impairment and increase production of amyloid β,[38] supporting the cholinergic theory. In addition, amyloid β has shown to interact with cholinergic receptors and reduce their function (► Fig. 5.2).[38]

5.5 Genetic Component of Alzheimer Disease

Both early-onset and late-onset AD have been linked to having a genetic predisposition.

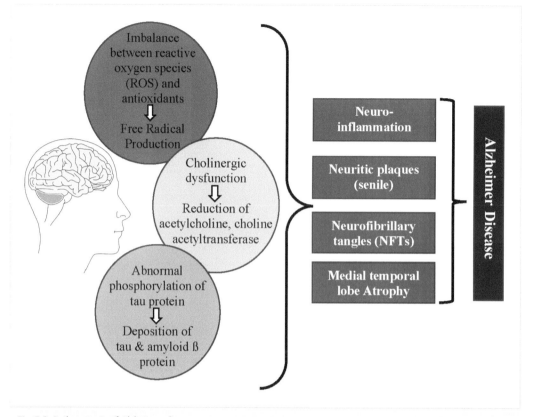

Fig. 5.2 Pathogenesis of Alzheimer disease.

5.5.1 Early Onset

Early-onset familial AD is an autosomal-dominant inheritance related to three genes: amyloid precursor protein (APP), presenilin 1 (PSEN-1), and presenilin 2 (PSEN-2).[4] This particular variant of the disease develops between the ages of 30 and 60 and attributes to less than 10% of all Alzheimer cases.[4] Early onset involves a single gene mutation on chromosomes 21, 14, and 1, resulting in abnormal protein formation.[45] APP, PSEN-1, and PSEN-2 mutations have been found to play a key role in APP breakdown, increasing the production of aggregation-prone forms of AB peptide that subsequently triggers the pathological process.[46,47,48]

Abnormal APP is located on chromosome 21. APP is a type 1 integral-membrane protein, concentrated in the synapses of neurons. Ten

to fifteen percent of the mutation of this protein occurs either in or next to the AB peptide sequence.[46] The AB peptide is the main constituent of amyloid plaques found in AD-affected brains.[46] Patients with Down syndrome (trisomy 21) have additionally been found to display neuropathological features of AD by the time they are in their forties, provided that they live that long.[4]

Presenilin-1 is a polytopic membrane protein and a component of the atypical aspartyl protease complex, which ultimately is liable for the cleavage of the AB peptide.[4] Mutations of this protein occur on chromosome 14 and are the most common causations of early-onset Alzheimer; studies have found this to be approximately 40 to 70%.[45] These mutations tend to cause an earlier age of onset, as early as 30 years old,[45] and the most severe form as a short yet rapid course of progression of the disease (6–7 years) compared with 11 years in PSEN-2.[46]

Alike PSEN-1, presenilin 2 is also a component of the atypical aspartyl protease complex.[4] PSEN-2 is found on chromosome 1 and mutations in this gene are an extremely rare cause of early-onset AD compared to PSEN-1, particularly in Caucasian populations.[4] Age of onset is variable among members of the same family that have been affected by this missense mutation; conversely, PSEN-1 causes relatively similar age of onset. It is unlikely that presenilin mutations will lead to late-onset AD.

5.5.2 Late Onset

Late-onset AD occurring around 60 to 65 years has a higher incidence, with more than 90% patients identified in this category.[4]

It is likely that genetics play an essential role with this type, however, only in conjunction with other lifestyle and environmental factors.[45] As yet, there has been no specific causative gene identified; however, having a form of the ApoE gene on chromosome 19 has been found to increase the risk of Alzheimer disease.[4,45,46] Associations with this gene have been linked to both sporadic and familial late-onset AD[4] and is vital in the pathogenesis of the disease.[45]

ApoE has different alleles including ApoE ε2, ApoE ε3, and ApoE ε4.[4] ApoE ε4 leads to inefficient amyloid clearance and is capable of producing toxic fragments once the molecule is cleaved.[4] ApoE ε4 falls into the category of a genetic risk-factor as it increases the risk of the development of AD, depending on the number of alleles a person has, the greatest being 2. However, this is not an accurate determination of the disease because some individuals expressing this allele do not present with AD, and, conversely, there are others who do not possess the ApoE ε4 allele but present with AD.[4] Thus, having this allele alone is not a necessary causative factor, yet it remains to be the most significant and well-established biological marker associated with late-onset

AD.[45] Having the ApoE ε2 allele is rare and may even have a reducing effect on the disease,[45] but if someone is found to have it, they are not likely to develop the disease until later in life.[4]

Genetic investigations have evolved considerably throughout the years, and ongoing research into the genetic components of AD is still being conducted. Recently, genome-wide association studies (GWAS) have found over 21 additional genetic risk loci to contribute to increased susceptibility of late-onset AD, supported by a sufficient level of evidence.[49,50,51] These include clusterin (CLU), phosphatidyl-inositol-binding clathrin assembly proteins (PICALM), exocyst complex component3-like 2 (EXOC3L2), bridging integrator 1 (BIN1), complement component receptor 1 (CR1), sortilin-related receptor (SORL1), nonreceptor tyrosine kinase 1 (TNK1), interleukin 8 (IL8), low-density lipoprotein receptor (LDLR), cystatin C (CST3), CHRNB2 gene (on chromosome 1), SORCS1, tumor necrosis factor alpha (TNF), chemokine receptor 2 (CCR2).[49] A number of these GWAS-identified risk genes are possibly linked with the AB cascade, but, notably, the majority of the associated genes accumulate within either of three pathways: endocytosis, inflammatory response, and cholesterol and lipid metabolism.[50,51] These risk genes emphasize the multifactorial nature of AD; however, they play a lesser role compared with ApoE gene, APP, PSEN-1, and PSEN-2.[49,50]

5.5.3 Genetic Testing

A blood test that identifies which APoE alleles a person has cannot be used with complete accuracy in diagnosing the possible development of AD for that particular individual. Also since there are other factors that contribute to the disease excluding genetics, it is unlikely that there will ever be a use of genetic testing in the prediction of development of the disease.[4,45,49] However, it does remain a good tool for studying AD risk in large groups of people. Genetic testing of the presenilins can be conducted, but it is only likely to reveal the early-onset AD, and therefore genetic counseling should be carried out in addition.[45]

5.6 Diagnostic Evaluation of Alzheimer Disease

5.6.1 Identification

Diagnosing AD is a multistep process, beginning with a thorough medical history that can include imaging procedures, neuropsychological testing, and other symptoms-dependent testing. Memory loss and cognitive decline are strongly indicative of Alzheimer disease.[52] The Mini-Mental State Examination (MMSE) is currently the most common tool in reaching an AD diagnosis. It consists of neuropsychological testing to identify issues with memory, language, planning, and attention span.[53] General questions such as "What is your name?," "What is the date?," and questions about living arrangements are asked. The Fuld Object Memory Test is also common in diagnosis.[54] Patients are shown ten objects, then asked to memorize the objects and repeat it to the examiner. Multiple cognitive deficits must be present to be diagnosed with AD. One deficit must be memory impairment. One study has put forward that patients with AD performed "significantly poorer on tests of short-term memory, temporal orientation, visual perception, and language,"[54] thus highlighting the importance of the MMSE and Fuld Object Memory Test as a means of diagnosis (▶ Fig. 5.3).

5.6.2 Medical History

A GP is often responsible for taking the patient's initial medical history. Guiding questions help in assessing risk factors for AD and the patient's ability to function in everyday life.[55] This process is often complicated by symptoms of the disease, that is, memory loss.[56] Having a family member present to describe the patient's condition and progression, as well as past medical history, is recommended. A history of the patient's medical problems such as a stroke, Parkinson disease, HIV infection, depression, a head injury, heart disease, or lipid disorders needs to be ascertained as these conditions can cause confusion or other signs of Alzheimer disease. In addition, the patient's family, social, cultural, and educational background are important, as these can influence how a person performs on a mental status test and other tests such as the Mini-Mental State Examination.[52] A history of substance abuse, mood changes, lack of inhibition, and issues with forgetfulness are important indicators for AD. In a study, severe headaches and migraine were inversely related to AD.[55] More cases than controls reported epilepsy before the onset of AD, especially for epilepsy with an onset within 10 years of AD.[55]

5.6.3 Physical Exam and Lab Testing

Along with a complete medical history, a physical exam is important in the evaluation of AD. Assessment of hearing, vision, blood pressure, pulse, and other basic indicators of health should be recorded. A physical exam can detect acute or chronic medical conditions such as an infection, chronic arterial hypertension, or chronic renal failure that might be causing confusion and other AD-like symptoms.[55] Cognitive testing and neurological exams such as evaluating speech and movement are common when AD is suspected. Neurological exams focus on an examination of the motor system, gait, functionality of reflexes, and coordination. Neuropsychological tests assess cognitive function through simple questionnaires that not only establish difficulties with memory but also track a change in the patient's cognitive difficulties over time. Along with these tests, brain imaging methods, such as single photon emission computed tomography (SPECT), computed tomography (CT) scan, positron emission tomography (PET) scan, or magnetic resonance imaging (MRI), are utilized.[57] In patients with AD symptoms, new brain imaging technology enables physicians to diagnose probable AD with almost 90% accuracy.[57] Unfortunately, the various diagnostic tests are only effective in diagnosing AD when a patient has already begun showing symptoms. This is problematic because the underlying causes of AD activate 10 to 20 years before any obvious symptoms

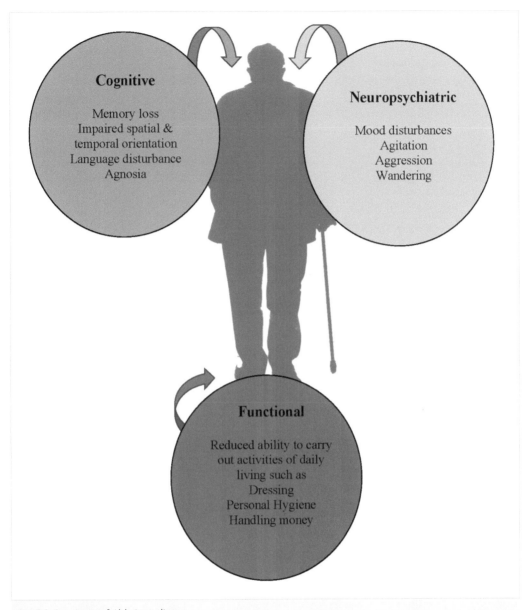

Fig. 5.3 Symptoms of Alzheimer disease.

of the disease appear.[54] Lab testing can be undertaken to compliment the physical exam and perceived symptoms. In addition to brain scans or electroencephalography that are often done, blood tests can be performed to investigate anemia, infection, electrolyte imbalance, liver function, vitamin B12 deficiency, and thyroid function, drug interactions and dosing problems. [56]

5.7 Medical Management and Treatment of Alzheimer Disease

Current therapeutic management of AD does not have the capacity to modify the course of the disease, which leads to a poor prognosis of the disease as there is no cure. Instead, management of AD is focused on relieving the symptoms and delaying the progression of the disease to provide a better quality of life for the individual.[58] The two universally accepted classes of drugs that are used to improve the symptoms of AD are cholinesterase inhibitors and N-methyl-D-aspartate receptor antagonist (NMDARA).

Cholinesterase inhibitors used in AD are centrally acting drugs such as donepezil, galantamine, and rivastigmine.[59] The mechanism of action of this class of drug is to deactivate the cholinesterase enzymes. With the inhibition of cholinesterase enzyme, the degradation of acetylcholine is blocked to maintain a high level of the acetylcholine within the synaptic cleft to induce activity on the remaining functional cholinergic synapses. The continual stimulation of cholinergic neurons will result in temporary improvement in cognitive functions as the cholinergic neurons are responsible for storage and processing of information.[60] However, cholinesterase inhibitors have been shown to be associated with nausea, hyper-salivation, syncope, fatigue, weight loss, and cardiovascular issues such as bradycardia, hypotension, and heart block.

The second class of drugs is N-Methyl-D-Aspartate Receptor antagonist such as memantine. This type of drug prevents the degradation of cholinergic neurons by preventing elevations in glutamate levels within the central nervous system. A high glutamate level in AD is caused by neuronal stimulation of beta-amyloid accumulation. The elevation in glutamate leads to overexcitation of the recipient neuron leading to excitotoxicity.[59] With the administration of NMDARA, the rate of cholinergic neuron degradation caused by excitotoxicity will be reduced to allow AD patient to maintain their cognitive function for a longer period of time. The potential side effects of Memantine are dizziness, blurred vision, and hypertension.[60]

According to Friedlander et al,[60] studies have been conducted in which vitamin E was incorporated into the AD medication which then resulted in a delayed development of dementia. The reason for this delay was hypothesized to be caused by the antioxidant property of vitamin E which provides a level of neuroprotection. However, if cholinesterase inhibitors and NMDARA are ineffective in the management of the individual's behavior, patients are prescribed antipsychotics, antidepressants, and mood stabilizers to control their behavior. With the use of central nervous system depressing drugs, there are many adverse effects that are relevant to oral health, such as xerostomia, stomatitis, dysgeusia, spasms of the muscle of mastication with the potential of causing temporomandibular joint dislocation, and potential candidal infections.[60] If the patient displays symptoms of adverse effects of the drugs used in the management of AD, the medication should be discontinued.

Currently, the development of disease-modifying drugs of AD is based on the amyloid hypothesis. These drugs aim to prevent the formation of beta-amyloid plaques by inhibiting beta and gamma secretase. By inhibiting either beta or gamma secretase, it will prevent the formation of beta-amyloid plaque from APP. Without the beta-amyloid plaque, impairment of synaptic function due to neurodegeneration will be limited to prevent further progression of AD. However, these drugs are currently still in clinical trials. The issue with secretase inhibitors is its nonspecific therapeutic effect as the secretases are also responsible for the cleavage of other proteins. Due to the nonspecific effects of the inhibitors, toxicity can result due to interference in the cell-to-cell interactions. Moreover, alpha-secretase activators are also undergoing development. Alpha-secretase will cleave the APP so that gamma-secretase can no longer cleave the protein to generate beta-amyloid.

Since NFTs are also an important element in the pathogenesis of AD along with the beta-amyloid plaque, potential future treatments can be aimed at inhibition of NFTs' formation. The formation of NFTs can be inhibited by the deactivation of glycogen synthase kinase 3β. This enzyme is responsible for the hyperphosphorylation of tau proteins to form the NFTs.[61] Another approach to the inhibition of NFTs' formation is to prevent the aggregation of tau proteins. According to Salmone et al,[59] methylthioninium chloride has shown to reduce beta-amyloid oligomerization, hence leading to a reduction in beta-amyloid plaque, and it occupies the domain on tau proteins which is responsible for aggregation. This compound has undergone phase 2b of clinical trials and demonstrated improvement in cognitive function of AD patient.

The control of behavior and maintenance of mental health in individuals with AD is an important aspect in the management of the disease. It has been shown that an ill mental health can contribute to the rapid decline in cognitive function.[62] The application of non-therapeutic interventions are methods in minimizing psychological signs and symptoms of AD. Studies have shown that cognitive therapy such as solving puzzles and simple arithmetic can improve the individual's mental capacity.[62] It is also important for patients with AD to maintain an active lifestyle and be socially active as it prevents the development of depression and an apathetic attitude. By maintaining an active lifestyle, it improves the quality of life and ensures that the individual can perform daily activities by themselves for a longer period of time. Furthermore, reminiscence therapy is another approach to improve the well-being of the patient in which the patients are encouraged to talk about their past. It has been shown that emotionally oriented therapy such as reminiscence therapy has a positive effect on mood and behavior.[62] Therefore, through the management of psychological and behavior issues present in Alzheimer patients, the individuals are more likely to experience a better quality of life.

5.8 Management of a Dental Patient with Alzheimer Disease

The consequences of cognitive-related conditions such as Alzheimer play a notable role in the management of patients and the development of a treatment plan in a dental setting. The increased incidence of tooth retention in the elderly as a result of effective preventative measures in adolescence and adulthood means that more complex management of Alzheimer patients is required than previous generations.

The close association between the existence of periodontal disease and progression of neurological dysfunction in AD patients indicates a close monitoring and treatment of the condition through root planning and subgingival scaling. Periodontal diseases are thought to hasten the cognitive condition through the increased production of proinflammatory cytokines during the diseased state or invasion of periopathogenic organisms through the blood–brain barrier.[63] Assisted bacterial clearance through the utilization of chemical plaque control agents may be indicated to reduce the risk of periodontal disease progression in Alzheimer patients capable of rinsing and spitting. This reduction in risk is related to penetration of the agent 1 to 2 mm subgingivally and decline in the apical migration of supra-gingival organisms. A chemical control agent of most benefit would be one that can be used long-term without any significant side effects, as well as exhibits appropriate antimicrobial properties. The mouthwash should preferably also contain fluoride to prevent the occurrence of root surface caries associated with gingival recession, which is a manifestation of a periodontal disease. Any restorative treatment required warrants careful consideration of the choice of restorative material, mainly due to current controversy concerning the relation between dental mercury and neurological disturbance.[64]

In the moderate-to-late stages of AD, there is only a paucity of muscle coordination remaining in concurrence with involuntary mouth movements, reducing denture retention and stability. These factors must be considered in the production of any prosthesis for such a patient, potentially indicating the use of products such as denture adhesives to attain an acceptable level of retention.[65] Reduced stability and retention of dentures in AD patients may be indicative of drug-induced xerostomia, indicating the need for saliva rate and quality assessment. Once identified, these individuals can be assisted through artificial saliva solutions.

The limited potential to accommodate an appropriate oral health regime indicates a need for dexterity assessments in patients with AD, and if insufficient, implement devices that require less dexterity, such as an electric toothbrush. In severe circumstances, it may be beneficial to designate the role of oral hygiene and denture maintenance to carers. These individuals need to be informed and guided by the dental professional on how to achieve an acceptable level of oral health in the patient. Reviews conducted have suggested a positive response with respect to oral hygiene maintenance in aged care facilities following the provision of comprehensive staff training.[66]

Agitation and aggression that is synonymous with certain cases of AD make routine dental procedures difficult to conduct. Such patients may require an extended allocation of time to ensure that patient care is delivered. Procedures that require immobilization including endodontic treatment may indicate the use of general anesthetics in a hospital setting, conditional to the severity of the neurological disorder. Sedation programs conducted have indicated the use of low-dose intravenous benzodiazepines with or without a barbiturate, subject to the degree of immobilization required.[67] The nature of AD is of particular concern when it comes to providing consent for dental procedures. Patients should, therefore, arrive with a statutory health attorney to permit the provision of care and patients capable of providing consent should be informed about advance health directives in case of disease advancement. A complete examination and assessment of the patient will determine the frequency of dental appointments, and if possible, the same dentist should be involved in the continuity of care for the patient to ensure effective and efficient treatment.

5.9 Oral Medicine Aspects of Alzheimer Disease

The manifestation of Alzheimer disease (AD) causes a variety of effects on the oral cavity, which result in a statistically significant reduction in oral health, reduce the efficacy of prosthetic appliances, and accelerate oral diseases.[68,69,70] The oral medicine relationship to Alzheimer disease has changed since the effectiveness of modern dental practice has allowed patients to maintain their dentition, previously it would be more common for them to become edentulous and have full upper and lower prostheses.[71] There has since been the argument that the focus should be on prevention and the maintenance of a healthy dentition since the costs associated with the oral medicine aspects of AD far outweigh those to maintain a clean healthy mouth.[72]

Multiple statistical analyses have been conducted to quantify the impact AD has on oral health.[68,69,73,74,75] Consistent findings indicate that denture hygiene and oral hygiene are compromised when compared to control groups of the same age as those with AD.[68] Furthermore, the risk of dental caries and periodontal disease is increased highest with AD of all the dementia categories in the study.[76] This was quantified through objective values of DMFT index (Decayed, Missing, and Filled Teeth) and OHI (Oral Health Index). The decline in oral hygiene was attributed to the deficits in cognitive and voluntary movement suffered by AD patients and showed a progressive trend as the disease advanced, which is consistent with prior studies.[74,77,78] Qualitative observation of patients found that 75% of patients with AD also presented with oral pathologies, most common of which was denture stomatitis.[68] In addition to reduced salivation from the anticholinergic action of some drugs,[78] false self-perception and cognitive deficits in AD patients result in neglect of the denture hygiene and consequently exacerbate the fungal infection as the oral cavity protection is now compromised.[79]

The nature of AD is such that drug therapies aimed at slowing the effects or progression of the disease also have a systemic interaction. Of particular relevance, given the mean age of AD patients being over 50,[71] is the effect these therapies have on the efficacy of prosthetic appliances. The treatment of AD is complex and often adjunctive medications are used such as antidepressants, benzodiazepines, and antipsychotics, which potentiate xerostomia increasing the possibility of ulcerations to the mucosa and inadequate retention of prosthetic appliances.[70] Conversely, choline esterase inhibitors are used to treat AD and potentiate salivation in their cholinergic action; patients may similarly experience difficulty in retaining prosthetic appliances; also they may pose a difficulty to practitioners in treatment due to difficulties in isolation and a choking hazard.[70]

Adjunctive drugs used in AD while often leading to xerostomia are accompanied by a general reduction in mucosal fluids, changing the normal flora existing in the mouth to one more conducive to the invasion of oral diseases including bacterial, viral, and fungal.[68] The specific effect this has reduces the flushing and buffering capacity of the mouth, leading to a reduced ability of the mouth to resist plaque formation and the proliferation of anaerobic bacteria.[70] The oral diseases conducive to this environment are gingivitis, periodontitis, dental caries, and retrograde infections causing sialadenitis.[80,81] Secondary effects from adjunctive treatment are also common, and one such treatment increases the risk of orofacial movement disorders. Haloperidol, while used less now in favor of those with fewer adverse effects, increases the risk of orofacial tardive dyskinesia that has associated complications of tooth wear, fracture, prosthesis damage, orofacial pain, TMJ degeneration, ulcers, chewing difficulties, dysphagia, weight loss, and social embarrassment due to their impediment.[80,82]

5.10 Coordination of Care between Dentist and Physician

Oral health is a major contributor to the overall well-being of Alzheimer patients, and thus coordination between the dentist and physician is paramount in the management of the disease. The additional needs of an Alzheimer patient should precipitate emphasis on treatment planning, especially in relation to the maintenance of dentition, promotion of a healthy diet, and monitoring symptom progression. Overall, coordination ensures a full understanding of clinical manifestations of the disease, resulting in safe and rational dental care.[83]

It is well documented that patients' oral health status and diet can have a significant influence on AD progression.[71] A recent study conducted on dental care utilization of dementia patients indicated that post-diagnosis, frequency of dental visits decreased (1.5 to 0.9 visits per year) while the prevalence of oral disease increased, resulting in greater tooth loss. It was widely admitted by participants that oral hygiene among patients and caregivers was often neglected, as patients have more prominent high-priority health issues. It was also concluded that individuals with severe mental impairment were three times more likely to be edentulous.[84] A diseased dentition impairs masticatory function, reducing consumption of raw foods and subsequently increasing intake of softer foods containing monounsaturated and polyunsaturated fatty acids, accelerating cognitive degeneration.[85] Although not curative, a collaborative approach of health care specialists promoting oral hygiene and nutrition can improve the overall prognosis for AD patients.

Adequate communication between physician and dentist also presents an opportunity to monitor drug side effects and adjust the course of treatment to meet patient requirements. Although the common drugs used to slow the progression of AD (galantamine, donepezil, and rivastigmine) are generally well tolerated, unfavorable side effects are experienced by a proportion of individuals.[86] In patients taking 6 to 12 mg/day rivastigmine plus memantine, the incidence of nausea and vomiting were 30 and 13%, respectively.[87] Long-term vomiting presents as macroscopic changes to the oral mucosa and enamel erosion, particularly on the palatal surface of upper incisors, which can be observed by the dentist during treatment.[88] In extension to the oral changes, continual exposure to gastric acids can result in an esophageal metaplasia–dysplasia transition, increasing the risk of esophageal adenocarcinoma.[89] Early diagnosis of cellular changes and intervention is essential as the disease has a 5-year survival rate of only 16%.[90] Side effects may not be readily communicated to the prescribing doctor by the patient or caregiver; however, symptoms can often be controlled, improving the patient's overall health.

Regular dental visits also facilitate monitoring patients' disease progression and ensuring adherence to medication. Although AD is recognized as a degenerative condition characterized by progressive impairment of cognitive function, a rapid deterioration in the patient's memory or behavioral changes between treatments is indicative of a lack of adherence or misuse of prescribed medications.[91] Through a collaborative approach, health professionals can maximize drug adherence and optimize the management of symptoms.

AD is an increasingly prevalent condition in the world's aging population that has many dental-related implications. Treatment options available for the condition have shown clinical success in terms of symptom improvement and cognitive function; however, they are not devoid of adverse effects. Compromised oral health as a result of cognitive dysfunction requires attention to avoid further progression of the condition and prevent the induction of other oral diseases related to neglected care. Strategies for effective management of AD patients are highly dependent on the severity of the condition. Family members and carers have a large role in the management of AD patients because of the inability to provide consent. Collaboration with other health professionals is imperative for awareness of drug interactions, formulation of treatment plans, and increasing the overall well-being of the patient.

References

[1] Winter Y, Korchounov A, Zhukova TV, Bertschi NE. Depression in elderly patients with Alzheimer dementia or vascular dementia and its influence on their quality of life. J Neurosci Rural Pract. 2011; 2(1):27–32

[2] Qiu C, Kivipelto M, von Strauss E. Epidemiology of Alzheimer's disease: occurrence, determinants, and strategies toward intervention. Dialogues Clin Neurosci. 2009; 11(2):111–128

[3] Toyota Y, Ikeda M, Shinagawa S, et al. Comparison of behavioral and psychological symptoms in early-onset and late-onset Alzheimer's disease. Int J Geriatr Psychiatry. 2007; 22(9):896–901

[4] Bekris LM, Yu CE, Bird TD, Tsuang DW. Genetics of Alzheimer disease. J Geriatr Psychiatry Neurol. 2010; 23(4):213–227

[5] Bookheimer S, Burggren A. APOE-4 genotype and neurophysiological vulnerability to Alzheimer's and cognitive aging. Annu Rev Clin Psychol. 2009; 5:343–362

[6] Robinson L, Tang E, Taylor JP. Dementia: timely diagnosis and early intervention. BMJ. 2015; 350:h3029

[7] Reisberg B, Ferris SH, de Leon MJ, et al. The stage specific temporal course of Alzheimer's disease: functional and behavioral concomitants based upon cross-sectional and longitudinal observation. Prog Clin Biol Res. 1989; 317:23–41

[8] Mueller SG, Weiner MW, Thal LJ, et al. Ways toward an early diagnosis in Alzheimer's disease: the Alzheimer's Disease Neuroimaging Initiative (ADNI). Alzheimers Dement. 2005; 1 (1):55–66

[9] Alzheimer's Association Report 2017.Alzheimer's disease facts and figures. Alzheimers Dement. 2017; 13:325–373

[10] Joshi A, Ringman JM, Lee AS, Juarez KO, Mendez MF. Comparison of clinical characteristics between familial and non-familial early onset Alzheimer's disease. J Neurol. 2012; 259(10):2182–2188

[11] Hippius H, Neundörfer G. The discovery of Alzheimer's disease. Dialogues Clin Neurosci. 2003; 5(1):101–108

[12] Brunnström HR, Englund EM. Cause of death in patients with dementia disorders. Eur J Neurol. 2009; 16(4):488–492

[13] Bassett DS, Gazzaniga MS. Understanding complexity in the human brain. Trends Cogn Sci. 2011; 15(5):200–209

[14] Mohamed T, Rao PP. Alzheimer's disease: emerging trends in small molecule therapies. Curr Med Chem. 2011; 18(28):4299–4320

[15] Kiernan JA. Anatomy of the temporal lobe. Epilepsy Research and Treatment. 2012; Article ID 176157

[16] Mosconi MW, Wang Z, Schmitt LM, Tsai P, Sweeney JA. The role of cerebellar circuitry alterations in the pathophysiology of autism spectrum disorders. Front Neurosci. 2015; 9:296

[17] Herculano-Houzel S. The human brain in numbers: a linearly scaled-up primate brain. Front Hum Neurosci. 2009; 3:31

[18] Lovinger DM. Communication networks in the brain. Alcohol Res Health. 2008; 31(3):196–214

[19] Maurer K, Volk S, Gerbaldo H. Auguste D and Alzheimer's disease. Lancet. 1997; 349(9064):1546–1549

[20] Schuff N, Woerner N, Boreta L, et al. Alzheimer's Disease Neuroimaging Initiative. MRI of hippocampal volume loss in early Alzheimer's disease in relation to ApoE genotype and biomarkers. Brain. 2009; 132(Pt 4):1067–1077

[21] Jahn H. Memory loss in Alzheimer's disease. Dialogues Clin Neurosci. 2013; 15(4):445–454

[22] Holtzman DM, Morris JC, Goate AM. Alzheimer's disease: the challenge of the second century. Sci Transl Med. 2011; 3(77):77sr1

[23] Zhang L, Zhou FM, Dani JA. Cholinergic drugs for Alzheimer's disease enhance in vitro dopamine release. Mol Pharmacol. 2004; 66(3):538–544

[24] Javaid FZ, Brenton J, Guo L, Cordeiro MF. Visual and ocular manifestations of Alzheimer's disease and their use as biomarkers for diagnosis and progression. Front Neurol. 2016; 7:55

[25] Liu CC, Liu CC, Kanekiyo T, Xu H, Bu G. Apolipoprotein E and Alzheimer disease: risk, mechanisms and therapy. Nat Rev Neurol. 2013; 9(2):106–118

[26] Chen JH, Lin KP, Chen YC. Risk factors for dementia. J Formos Med Assoc. 2009; 108(10):754–764

[27] Grill JD, Cummings JL. Novel targets for Alzheimer's disease treatment. Expert Rev Neurother. 2010; 10(5):711–728

[28] Takeda M, Tanaka T, Okochi M, Kazui H. Non-pharmacological intervention for dementia patients. Psychiatry Clin Neurosci. 2012; 66(1):1–7

[29] Rolim TdS, Fabri GM, Nitrini R, et al. Evaluation of patients with Alzheimer's disease before and after dental treatment. Arq Neuropsiquiatr. 2014; 72(12):919–924

[30] Abbayya K, Puthanakar NY, Naduwinmani S, Chidambar YS. Association between periodontitis and Alzheimer's disease. N Am J Med Sci. 2015; 7(6):241–246

[31] Kamer AR, Fortea JO, Videla S, et al. Periodontal disease's contribution to Alzheimer's disease progression in Down syndrome. Alzheimers Dement (Amst). 2016; 2:49–57

[32] Alzheimer's Association. 2016 Alzheimer's disease facts and figures. Alzheimers Dement. 2016; 12(4):459–509

[33] Aschenbrenner AJ, Balota DA, Gordon BA, Ratcliff R, Morris JC. A diffusion model analysis of episodic recognition in preclinical individuals with a family history for Alzheimer's disease: the adult children study. Neuropsychology. 2016; 30 (2):225–238

[34] Niu H, Álvarez-Álvarez I, Guillén-Grima F, Aguinaga-Ontoso I. Prevalence and incidence of Alzheimer's disease in Europe: a meta-analysis. Neurologia. 2017; 32(8):523–532

[35] Chen C-K, Wu Y-T, Chang Y-C. Association between chronic periodontitis and the risk of Alzheimer's disease: a retrospective, population-based, matched-cohort study. Alzheimers Res Ther. 2017; 9(1):56

[36] Solomon A, Mangialasche F, Richard E, et al. Advances in the prevention of Alzheimer's disease and dementia. J Intern Med. 2014; 275(3):229–250

[37] Swerdlow RH. Pathogenesis of Alzheimer's disease. Clin Interv Aging. 2007; 2(3):347–359

[38] Sanabria-Castro A, Alvarado-Echeverría I, Monge-Bonilla C. Molecular pathogenesis of Alzheimer's disease: an update. Ann Neurosci. 2017; 24(1):46–54

[39] Tudorache IF, Trusca VG, Gafencu AV, Apolipoprotein E. Apolipoprotein E-A multifunctional protein with implications in various pathologies as a result of its structural features. Comput Struct Biotechnol J. 2017; 15:359–365

[40] Kara E, Marks JD, Fan Z, et al. Isoform- and cell type-specific structure of apolipoprotein E lipoparticles as revealed by a novel Forster resonance energy transfer assay. J Biol Chem. 2017; 292(36):14720–14729

[41] Kasper D, Fauci A, Hauser S, McGraw Hill C. Harrison's Principles of Internal Medicine. 19th ed. New York: McGraw-Hill Professional Publishing; 2015

[42] Puzzo D, Piacentini R, Fá M, et al. LTP and memory impairment caused by extracellular Aβ and Tau oligomers is APP-dependent. eLife. 2017; 6:6

[43] Theendakara V, Bredesen DE, Rao RV. Downregulation of protein phosphatase 2A by apolipoprotein E: implications for Alzheimer's disease. Mol Cell Neurosci. 2017; 83:83–91

[44] Mukhin VN. The role of the basal forebrain cholinergic dysfunction in pathogenesis of declarative memory disorder in Alzheimer's disease. Ross Fiziol Zh Im I M Sechenova. 2013; 99(6):674–681

[45] Braunwald E, Fauci A, Kasper D, Hauser S, Longo D, Jameson L. Harrison's Principles of Internal Medicine. 11th ed. New York: McGraw-Hill Book Company; 2001

[46] Cacace R, Sleegers K, Van Broeckhoven C. Molecular genetics of early-onset Alzheimer's disease revisited. Alzheimers Dement. 2016; 12(6):733–748

[47] Kikuchi K, Kidana K, Tatebe T, Tomita T. Dysregulated metabolism of the amyloid β protein and therapeutic approaches in Alzheimer disease. J Cell Biochem. 2017; 118(12):4183–4190

[48] Nicolas G, Charbonnier C, Campion D. From common to rare variants: the genetic component of Alzheimer disease. Hum Hered. 2016; 81(3):129–141

[49] Olgiati P, Politis AM, Papadimitriou GN, De Ronchi D, Serretti A. Genetics of late-onset Alzheimer's disease: update from the Alzgene database and analysis of shared pathways. Int J Alzheimers Dis. 2011; 2011:832379

[50] Van Cauwenberghe C, Van Broeckhoven C, Sleegers K. The genetic landscape of Alzheimer disease: clinical implications and perspectives. Genet Med. 2016; 18(5):421–430

[51] Giri M, Zhang M, Lü Y. Genes associated with Alzheimer's disease: an overview and current status. Clin Interv Aging. 2016; 11:665–681

[52] Terry RD, Masliah E, Salmon DP, et al. Physical basis of cognitive alterations in Alzheimer's disease: synapse loss is the major correlate of cognitive impairment. Ann Neurol. 1991; 30(4):572–580

[53] Galasko D, Klauber MR, Hofstetter CR, Salmon DP, Lasker B, Thal LJ. The Mini-Mental State Examination in the early diagnosis of Alzheimer's disease. Arch Neurol. 1990; 47(1):49–52

[54] Eslinger PJ, Damasio AR, Benton AL, Van Allen M. Neuropsychologic detection of abnormal mental decline in older persons. JAMA. 1985; 253(5):670–674

[55] Breteler MM, van Duijn CM, Chandra V, et al. EURODEM Risk Factors Research Group. Medical history and the risk of Alzheimer's disease: a collaborative re-analysis of case-control studies. Int J Epidemiol. 1991; 20 Suppl 2:S36–S42

[56] Coyle JT, Price DL, DeLong MR. Alzheimer's disease: a disorder of cortical cholinergic innervation. Science. 1983; 219 (4589):1184–1190

[57] DeKosky ST, Shih W-J, Schmitt FA, Coupal J, Kirkpatrick C. Assessing utility of single photon emission computed tomography (SPECT) scan in Alzheimer disease: correlation with cognitive severity. Alzheimer Dis Assoc Disord. 1990; 4(1):14–23

[58] Gregori M, Masserini M, Mancini S. Nanomedicine for the treatment of Alzheimer's disease. Nanomedicine (Lond). 2015; 10(7):1203–1218

[59] Danysz W, Parsons CG. Alzheimer's disease, β-amyloid, glutamate, NMDA receptors and memantine: searching for the connections. Br J Pharmacol. 2012; 167(2):324–352

[60] Friedlander AH, Norman DC, Mahler ME, Norman KM, Yagiela JA. Alzheimer's disease: psychopathology, medical management and dental implications. J Am Dent Assoc. 2006; 137 (9):1240–1251

[61] Salomone S, Caraci F, Leggio GM, Fedotova J, Drago F. New pharmacological strategies for treatment of Alzheimer's disease: focus on disease modifying drugs. Br J Clin Pharmacol. 2012; 73(4):504–517

[62] Grossberg GT, Desai AK. Management of Alzheimer's disease. J Gerontol A Biol Sci Med Sci. 2003; 58(4):331–353

[63] Allen GI, Amoroso N, Anghel C, et al. Alzheimer's Disease Neuroimaging Initiative. Crowdsourced estimation of cognitive decline and resilience in Alzheimer's disease. Alzheimers Dement. 2016; 12(6):645–653

[64] Mutter J, Naumann J, Schneider R, Walach H. Mercury and Alzheimer's disease. Fortschr Neurol Psychiatr. 2007; 75(9):528–538

[65] Kumar PR, Shajahan PA, Mathew J, Koruthu A, Aravind P, Ahammed MF. Denture adhesives in prosthodontics: an overview. J Int Oral Health. 2015; 7 Suppl 1:93–95

[66] Pearson A, Chalmers J. Oral hygiene care for adults with dementia in residential aged care facilities. JBI Library Syst Rev. 2004; 2(3):1–89

[67] Malamed SF, Gottschalk HW, Mulligan R, Quinn CL. Intravenous sedation for conservative dentistry for disabled patients. Anesth Prog. 1989; 36(4–5):140–142

[68] Ribeiro GR, Costa JL, Ambrosano GM, Garcia RC. Oral health of the elderly with Alzheimer's disease. Oral Surg Oral Med Oral Pathol Oral Radiol. 2012; 114(3):338–343

[69] Syrjälä AM, Ylöstalo P, Ruoppi P, et al. Dementia and oral health among subjects aged 75 years or older. Gerodontology. 2012; 29(1):36–42

[70] Turner LN, Balasubramaniam R, Hersh EV, Stoopler ET. Drug therapy in Alzheimer disease: an update for the oral health care provider. Oral Surg Oral Med Oral Pathol Oral Radiol Endod. 2008; 106(4):467–476

[71] Foltyn P. Ageing, dementia and oral health. Aust Dent J. 2015; 60 Suppl 1:86–94

[72] Hurd MD, Martorell P, Delavande A, Mullen KJ, Langa KM. Monetary costs of dementia in the United States. N Engl J Med. 2013; 368(14):1326–1334

[73] Turner MD, Ship JA. Dry mouth and its effects on the oral health of elderly people. J Am Dent Assoc. 2007; 138 Suppl: 15S–20S

[74] Ship JA. Oral health of patients with Alzheimer's disease. J Am Dent Assoc. 1992; 123(1):53–58

[75] Ship JA, Puckett SA. Longitudinal study on oral health in subjects with Alzheimer's disease. J Am Geriatr Soc. 1994; 42(1):57–63

[76] Warren JJ, Chalmers JM, Levy SM, Blanco VL, Ettinger RL. Oral health of persons with and without dementia attending a geriatric clinic. Spec Care Dentist. 1997; 17(2):47–53

[77] Adam H, Preston AJ. The oral health of individuals with dementia in nursing homes. Gerodontology. 2006; 23(2):99–105

[78] Mancini M, Grappasonni I, Scuri S, Amenta F. Oral health in Alzheimer's disease: a review. Curr Alzheimer Res. 2010; 7(4):368–373

[79] Kocaelli H, Yaltirik M, Yargic LI, Özbas H. Alzheimer's disease and dental management. Oral Surg Oral Med Oral Pathol Oral Radiol Endod. 2002; 93(5):521–524

[80] Boyce HW, Bakheet MR. Sialorrhea: a review of a vexing, often unrecognized sign of oropharyngeal and esophageal disease. J Clin Gastroenterol. 2005; 39(2):89–97

[81] Somerman MJ. Dental implications of pharmacological management of the Alzheimer's patient. Gerodontology. 1987; 6(2):59–66

[82] Daiello LA. Atypical antipsychotics for the treatment of dementia-related behaviors: an update. Med Health R I. 2007; 90(6):191–194

[83] Henry RG, Smith BJ. Managing older patients who have neurologic disease: Alzheimer disease and cerebrovascular accident. Dent Clin North Am. 2009; 53(2):269–294, ix

[84] Fereshtehnejad SM, Garcia-Ptacek S, Religa D, et al. Dental care utilization in patients with different types of dementia: a longitudinal nationwide study of 58,037 individuals. Alzheimers Dement. 2018; 14(1):10–19

[85] Solfrizzi V, Custodero C, Lozupone M, et al. Relationships of dietary patterns, foods, and micro- and macronutrients with Alzheimer's disease and late-life cognitive disorders: a systematic review. J Alzheimers Dis. 2017; 59(3):815–849

[86] Caraci F, Sultana J, Drago F, Spina E. Clinically relevant drug interactions with anti-Alzheimer's drugs. CNS Neurol Disord Drug Targets. 2017; 16(4):501–513

[87] Olin JT, Bhatnagar V, Reyes P, Koumaras B, Meng X, Brannan S. Safety and tolerability of rivastigmine capsule with memantine in patients with probable Alzheimer's disease: a 26-week, open-label, prospective trial (Study ENA713B US32). Int J Geriatr Psychiatry. 2010; 25(4):419–426

[88] Paszyńska EM, Słopień A, Osińska A, Dmitrzak-Węglarz M, Rajewski A, Surdacka A. Changes in oral cavity during period of intensive vomiting in patient with somatoform autonomic dysfunction: description of the case. Psychiatr Pol. 2016; 50(3):521–531

[89] Shivappa N, Hebert JR, Anderson LA, et al. Dietary inflammatory index and risk of reflux oesophagitis, Barrett's oesophagus and oesophageal adenocarcinoma: a population-based case-control study. Br J Nutr. 2017; 117(9):1323–1331

[90] Hopper AD, Campbell JA. Early diagnosis of oesophageal cancer improves outcomes. Practitioner. 2016; 260(1791):23–28, 3

[91] Pasqualetti G, Tognini S, Calsolaro V, Polini A, Monzani F. Potential drug-drug interactions in Alzheimer patients with behavioral symptoms. Clin Interv Aging. 2015; 10:1457–1466

6 Stroke

Armin Ariana

Abstract

Stroke as the second leading cause of death after ischemic heart disease is a preventable and treatable disease; however, it has become a global epidemic of the 21st century. Inadequate delivery of blood supply to the brain causes the cerebrovascular accident or stroke and can potentially lead to functional impairments, severe brain damage, and, consequently, death. Common long-term effects include contralateral limb paralysis, memory loss, and cognitive impairment. The introduction of brain imaging technology has revolutionized the diagnosis of stroke. This has been followed by a gradual decrease in the occurrence of stroke in developed countries; however, it is still a burden in low- and middle-income countries. Due to the limited effectiveness of stroke treatment options, the main approach for stroke management has become secondary prevention. This strategy focuses on controlling risk factors such as hypertension, high LDL cholesterol levels, and diabetes. The range in orofacial clinical manifestations of stroke is determined by size and location of the affected brain region. The most prevalent signs and symptoms include sensory and motor deficits: facial droop, paresis in extraocular muscles and eye movements, slurred speech, seizures, and neurocognitive deficits. Because of the potential adverse drug reactions, it is crucial that prior to any surgical or procedure treatment, close collaboration between health practitioners occurs to assess the bleeding risks of continued anticoagulant medication against the risk of post-thrombosis in ceasing anticoagulant medication.

Keywords: stroke, epidemiology, pathogenesis, oral manifestations, medical management, treatment

6.1 Background of Stroke

Despite being a preventable and treatable disease, stroke has become a global epidemic of the 21st century. In 2010, an estimated 16.9 million stroke incidents occurred, of which 5.9 million lives were lost; this makes stroke the second leading cause of death after ischemic heart disease.[1] Caused by an inadequate blood supply to the brain, cerebrovascular accident or stroke can potentially lead to functional impairments, severe brain damage, and, consequently, death.[2] Common long-term effects include contralateral limb paralysis, memory loss, and cognitive impairment.[2]

Evidence accumulated over the past 20 years has negated the conventional perception of stroke as merely a consequence of aging.[3] In the 1970s, evidence showed that aspirin could prevent stroke, followed by the establishment of the first stroke unit in 1975 and subsequently, the introduction of brain imaging technology, which has revolutionized stroke diagnosis.[3] Although there has been a gradual decrease in stroke occurrence in developed countries, 85% of the global burden of stroke is carried by low- and middle-income countries.[4] This has led current research to steer more toward further effective primary and secondary prevention strategies, cooperation among major government and nongovernment stakeholders, and incorporation of stroke management education and training for healthcare professionals.[4]

Due to the limited effectiveness of stroke treatment options, the main approach for stroke management has become secondary prevention. This strategy focuses on controlling risk factors such as hypertension, high LDL cholesterol levels, and diabetes.[5]

This chapter discusses the diagnosis, epidemiology, pathological, and genetic factors, as well as current available medical and dental treatment and prevention strategies of cerebrovascular accidents.

6.2 Description of Stroke

Stroke is defined as an "acute episode of focal disturbance of cerebral function" that lasts longer than 24 hours or of any duration if "diagnostic imaging shows any focal haemorrhage."[1]

There are two major classifications of stroke: ischemic stroke and hemorrhagic stroke.

6.2.1 Ischemic Stroke

Eighty-five percent of strokes are ischemic, which is caused by abrupt blockage of a cerebral artery leading to insufficient blood supply to a part of the brain.[2] Ischemic strokes can be classified as thrombotic or embolic. Thrombotic strokes are caused by a blood clot (thrombus) formation that blocks an artery supplying blood to the brain.[2] In embolic strokes, the blood clot is carried from another part of the body through the bloodstream to the brain, where it is lodged in the arteries.[2]

6.2.2 Hemorrhagic Stroke

A hemorrhagic stroke occurs due to the rupture of a blood vessel in the brain, causing bleeding in the surrounding tissue.[6] Due to the increased blood pressure inside the artery, as it bursts, it may potentially damage the surrounding tissue.[6] This results in a larger clot that places pressure on the brain, ultimately causing brain death. There are two main subtypes of hemorrhagic stroke, intracerebral and subarachnoid.[6]

In an intracerebral hemorrhage (ICH), bleeding within the brain exerts pressure on the surrounding tissues.[6] Common causes include high blood pressure, bleeding disorders, and blood vessel deformities such as aneurysm. In the subarachnoid hemorrhage (SAH), a blood vessel on the surface of the brain ruptures, and the blood from the ruptured vessel accumulates in the subarachnoid space.[6] Due to the blood build-up, pressure within the space increases, causing a common symptom of SAH called "thunderclap headache," one of the most severe headaches described by patients.[6]

Transient ischemic attacks are strokelike episodes (having the same symptoms) that last for a short time, usually within 24 hours.[2]

6.3 Epidemiology of Stroke

Cerebrovascular accident (stroke) was the third leading cause of death in 2015.[7] In 2015, fifteen million people worldwide suffered from stroke; 5 million of these cases passed away while 5 million were left with permanent disability.[5] It was estimated, in 2001, that the number of deaths attributed to stroke was approximately 5.5 million worldwide. Two-thirds of these deaths occurred in developing countries, and the subjects were less than 70 years old in 40% of these deaths.[8] Over 80% of strokes occur in people aged 65 years and older.[9] Stroke was the cause of 9.4% of deaths in Australia in 2001. On top of these mortality figures, stroke is also a leading global cause of permanent disability. In 2001, cerebrovascular disease contributed 2.2% of the morbidity rate in people aged 55 and older.[10] The burden of stroke is estimated to increase from 38 million disability-adjusted life years (DALYs) in 2000 to 61 million DALYs in 2020.[5] The average age when stroke occurs in developed countries is approximately 73 years, and it may be associated with the aging population within these countries. However, in developing countries, the average age of stroke occurrence is younger, due to different competing causes of death in these countries, such as communicable disease.[8] It has been reported that in countries with a higher gross domestic product (GDP) per capita, women and men experience cardiovascular events, such as stroke, at an older age than those with a lower GDP per capita.[11]

The prevalence of each type of stroke is seen to vary between different populations. For example, studies in the 1990s in Caucasian populations found that approximately 80% of strokes are ischemic, while 10 to 15% were ICH and 5% SAH. The remaining percentages were due to other causes of stroke. On the other hand, studies in Asian populations have indicated a higher incidence of ICH causing 20 to 30% of all strokes in those countries.[8] In addition, ICH has been demonstrated as the most fatal form of stroke in the United States, causing the highest proportion of in-hospital mortality due to stroke between 1997 and 2006.[12] Following coronary heart disease, stroke was considered the second highest cause of mortality due to cardiovascular disease in the United States in 2007.[12]

In 2015, stroke was the third leading cause of years of life lost (YLLs), whereas it was the fifth leading cause of YLLs in 2000.[7] The average YLLs due to stroke around the world was similar for males and females, at approximately 6 years per 1,000 men and women in 2000.[8]

Important risk factors for stroke include hypertension, body mass index (BMI), age, and blood cholesterol concentration.[13] Tobacco use is also an important modifiable risk factor.[14] Hypertension is closely associated with the development and severity of a stroke attack. Individuals who suffer from hypertension are more susceptible to stroke, as it predisposes atherosclerosis that promotes the formation of a cerebral embolism in the event of plaque rupture.[9] It can also be seen that alterations in vasculature with age render individuals more susceptible to the damaging effects of cardiovascular diseases, including stroke. The risk of stroke doubles for every 7.5 mm Hg increase in the diastolic blood pressure, and thus, the use of different antihypertensives have been shown to reduce the risk of stroke by 38%.[15] These risk factors have been proven by findings in cohorts of women and men in the United States, which have recognized that individuals with a healthier lifestyle: abstaining from smoking, participating in regular exercise, moderate alcohol consumption, and not being overweight, contributed to approximately an 80% lower risk of ischemic stroke compared to individuals not participating in any of these healthier behaviors.[11]

Most of the risk factors for cerebrovascular accident can be classified into inherent biological traits, behaviors, and social, environmental, and medical factors. Examples of inherent biological traits include age, sex, and physiological characteristics such as blood cholesterol levels and blood pressure whereas behavior encompasses diet and physical activity. Social factors such as education and ethnicity, and environmental factors including altitude and temperature, geographical or psychosocial environments, can also contribute to the risk of stroke. Medical factors, such as previous stroke, ischemic heart disease, atrial fibrillation, carotid stenosis, cardiovascular diseases, or glucose intolerance, are also important indicators that can predispose the development of stroke.[8]

6.3.1 Etiology and Pathogenesis of Stroke

Cerebrovascular accident (stroke) is of multifactorial etiology, which is why the pathogenesis of ischemic stroke is closely associated with multiple risk factors, including hypertension, atherosclerosis, and hyperlipidemia (▶ Fig. 6.1). The most common cause of ischemic stroke is the narrowing of arteries within the head and neck.[16] On the other hand, the pathogenesis of ICH involves degenerative changes within smooth muscle and endothelial cells.[17]

Hypertension promotes the formation of atherosclerotic plaques within medium-to-large arteries and microatheroma in smaller arteries. As a chronic disease directly influenced by diet, atherosclerosis can cause a high degree of arterial stenosis that leads to ischemic stroke symptoms. The narrowing of smaller arteries can also be emphasized due to the proliferation of endothelial cells and the hypertrophy of smooth muscles.[18] Plaques that are the most vulnerable to rupture are built of a large lipid core, composed of more than 40% low-density lipoprotein-filled foam cells, as well as a thin, fibrous cap of depleted smooth muscle cells. Macrophage infiltration is as well a characteristic of atherosclerotic

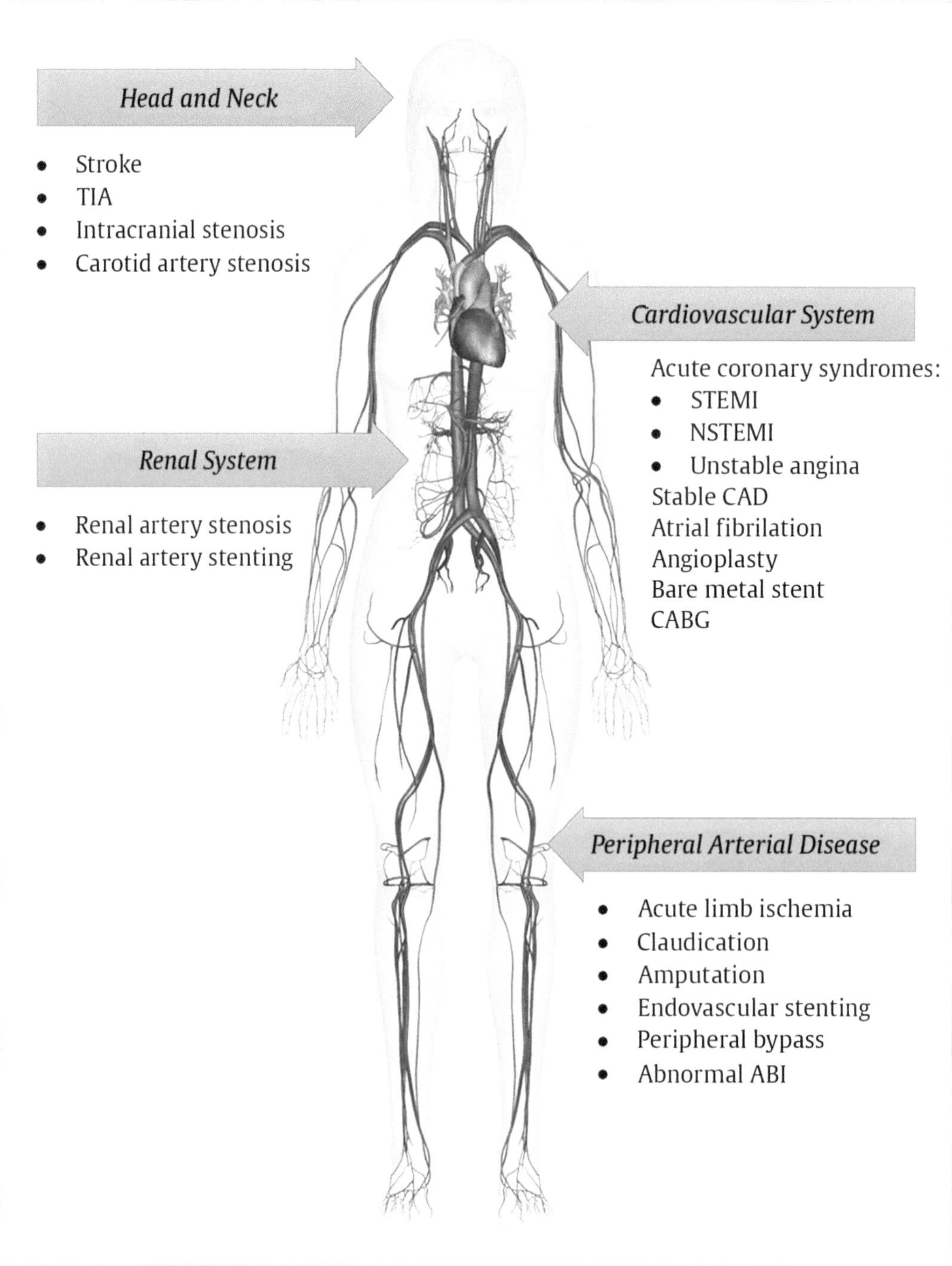

Head and Neck

- Stroke
- TIA
- Intracranial stenosis
- Carotid artery stenosis

Cardiovascular System

Acute coronary syndromes:
- STEMI
- NSTEMI
- Unstable angina

Stable CAD
Atrial fibrilation
Angioplasty
Bare metal stent
CABG

Renal System

- Renal artery stenosis
- Renal artery stenting

Peripheral Arterial Disease

- Acute limb ischemia
- Claudication
- Amputation
- Endovascular stenting
- Peripheral bypass
- Abnormal ABI

Fig. 6.1 Etiology of stroke.

plaques, contributing to the vulnerability of the plaque to rupture.[16]

Furthermore, small noncoding microRNAs (miRNAs) have been showed to contribute to stroke etiology. miRNA can modulate the pathogenesis of atherosclerosis (miR-21, miR-26), hyperlipidemia (miR-33, miR-125a-5p), hypertension (miR-15), and plaque rupture (miR-222, miR-210), which are all risk factors for the development of stroke. miRNA directs macrophage recruitment to atheromatous plaque vascular adhesion molecule-1 (VCAM1), expressed in human conditions, which promotes atherosclerosis formation. The decreased expression of miR-126 upregulates VCAM1 expression that enhances leukocyte adherence to the vascular endothelium. This, thereby, leads to leaky vessels, hemorrhage, partial embryonic lethality due to the loss of vascular integrity, and defects in endothelial cell proliferation, migration, and angiogenesis.[16]

When considering changes in the blood vessel lumen, it is also important to consider adaptive structural changes relating to resistance within the vessel. When hypertension occurs, collateral blood vessels adapt via increasing the total peripheral resistance and, as a consequence, compromise the collateral circulation. This thus increases the risk of ischemic events such as stroke in connection with the hypotension occurring distal to the stenosis.[17]

Although there is a clear link that stroke is the manifestation of hypertension, atherosclerosis, and other cardiovascular diseases, the pathogenesis of stroke can also be as a result of the interactions of genes with environmental determinants. For example, a link has been made between the pathogenesis of multifactorial forms of stroke and genes that encode hormones affecting the cardiovascular system such as atrial natriuretic peptide (ANP).[19]

6.4 Genetic Component of Stroke

Cerebrovascular accidents are considered to be a syndrome, rather than a single disease, with its onset being primarily attributed to preexisting conditions. Obesity, diabetes, atrial fibrillation, coronary heart disease, and cholesterol are examples of risk factors and account for up to 60% of stroke cases. The other 40% of risk factors are of either an unknown origin or attributed to rare genetic mutations, which are categorized into single or polygenic disorders.[20] When referring to strokes as a cause of genetic factors, this encompasses the manifestation of contributing predisposing diseases as well as hereditary stroke syndromes.

6.5 Predisposing Disease

6.5.1 Atrial Fibrillation

Atrial fibrillation, a type of arrhythmia, is considered to be a contributing factor and therefore sufferers are at a greater risk for the development of a stroke. Genome-wide association studies have concluded that atrial fibrillation is the most frequent cause of cardioembolic stroke, a subtype of ischemic stroke. In addition, no other significant relationships were determined between atrial fibrillation and other stroke subtypes. Two genes have been identified in which mutations are associated with atrial fibrillation, gene *PITX2* on 4q25, and gene *ZFHX3* on 16q22.[21]

Coronary Artery Disease and Associated Diseases

Coronary artery disease has shown to be associated with large-artery stroke; this correlation is attributed to single nucleotide polymorphism (SNPs) of the chromosome region 9p21.[22] Interestingly, mutations along the same locus have also been associated with intracranial and abdominal aneurysms, both of which are risk factors for strokes. Genes on this locus include *CDK2MA* and *CDK2MB*, variants of these genes are noncoding DNA sequences, an indication that mutations are determined by influences on gene expression.[21]

Single-Gene Disorder—Cerebral Autosomal Dominant Arteriopathy with Subcortical Infarcts and Leukoencephalopathy (CADASIL)

CADASIL is a single-gene disorder, in which its mode of inheritance is autosomal dominant. Of the monogenic disorders, CADASIL is the most common form of small vessel disease stroke. Offspring that present with this condition are characterized by deterioration of vascular smooth muscles cells. This is followed by arteriopathy causing impaired blood flow accompanied by blurred vision, migraines, and epilepsy. The reduction of blood flow in. the brain induces infarcts in 70% of CADASIL cases; recurrent strokes are also common.[23]

CADASIL is thought to be the result of a mutation of the gene NOTCH3, which is essential for the regulation of blood vessel health. Pathogenic mutations of NOTCH3 have shown to increase the deposition of cysteine within the blood vessels, due to an increase of this amino acid in the extracellular domain of NOTCH3.[21] However, little is known about the significance of this accumulation. Other studies have suggested that a defective NOTCH3 gene causes the accumulation of granular osmiophilic material within the vessels of the brain, damaging the white matter and obstructing blood flow.[24]

Among individuals with CADASIL, including family members, there is a high degree of phenotypic variation. Therefore, utilizing genotypes does not provide an accurate representation of an individual's phenotype.[25] Disparities among sufferers include the age of stroke onset, disease development, and prognosis.

Polygenic Disorder—Homocysteinemia

Homocysteinemia is an autosomal recessive inherited condition, which is characterized by elevated blood homocysteine levels. As it is a polygenic-induced condition, an interplay between various genetic and environmental factors is necessary for phenotypes to be expressed. Consequences of a marked increase in homocysteine levels can lead to the development of carotid stenosis, along with increased plaque thickness within the carotid artery. Therefore, homocysteinemia is a causative factor contributing to the manifestation of a stroke (large- and small-vessel disease subtype).[21]

Hyperhomocysteinemia cases are primarily the cause of abnormal metabolism of methionine; this is exacerbated by factors such as vitamin B12 and folate deficiencies along with renal failure.[26] Homocysteine levels are governed by the genes methylene-tetrahydrofolate reductase (MTHFR) and cystathionine-beta synthase (CbS); thus, polymorphism of these genes is associated with varied homocysteine levels. Common mutations include substitution of the gene responsible for encoding MTHFR, c.677C4T, as well as nucleotide variation of c.833C4T and c.919G4A on the CbS gene. More than 60 mutations related to both CbS and MTHFR genes have been discovered, resulting in moderate hyperhomocysteinemia.[26]

The genetic causes of strokes are extensive, many of which are unknown and require additional research. Despite the few examples listed in this chapter, a vast array of gene disorders contribute to its manifestation. This serves to emphasize the complexity, modes of inheritance, and genes involved as causative factors for the development of a stroke.

6.6 Diagnostic Evaluation of Stroke

6.6.1 Identification

Individuals who undergo cerebrovascular accidents will display various cardinal symptoms. These include drooping of the face, arm weakness, numbness, and speech impairments.[27] A stroke can be the cause of disruption to the nervous system; thus, an onset may occur sporadically, and symptoms may present contralateral to the side of the injury.[27] Other immediate identifying features include confusion, memory loss, paralysis of the body, headache, and vision impairment.[27]

6.6.2 Medical History

Various factors and conditions contribute to the manifestation of a stroke; therefore, utilizing the patient's medical history can serve as a good indicator of their risk. Diabetes, hypertension, heart disease, and the level of physical activity are identifiable risk factors.[28] Other important factors that are considered are the duration and cause of symptoms or any prescribed medications. Existing cardiovascular conditions such as atherosclerosis and atrial fibrillation are also of importance as they are predisposing diseases that may result in an ischemic stroke.[28]

6.6.3 Physical Examination

An impaired neurological function is typically seen in patients who are at risk for the development of a stroke (▶ Fig. 6.2). Therefore, mental capacity, cognition, as well as gait and

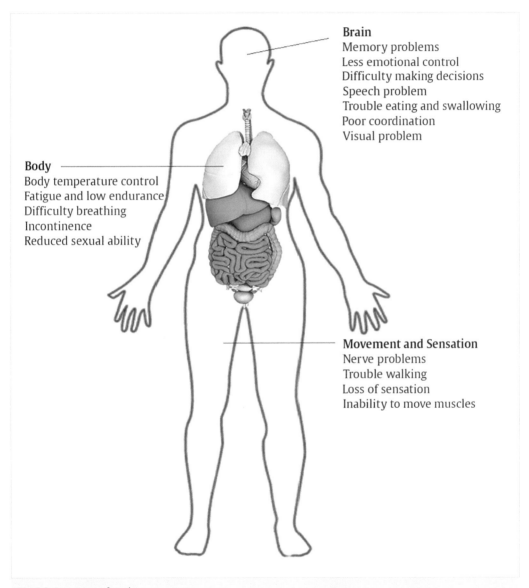

Fig. 6.2 Symptoms of stroke.

Brain
Memory problems
Less emotional control
Difficulty making decisions
Speech problem
Trouble eating and swallowing
Poor coordination
Visual problem

Body
Body temperature control
Fatigue and low endurance
Difficulty breathing
Incontinence
Reduced sexual ability

Movement and Sensation
Nerve problems
Trouble walking
Loss of sensation
Inability to move muscles

coordination are examined.[27] In addition, assessing whether the patient is able to raise their arms without contralateral deviation, and contracting their facial muscles, gives an indication of muscular weakness. Auscultation of the heart using a stethoscope may be performed to hear any carotid bruit as a sign of atherosclerosis.[27] Furthermore, an ophthalmoscope can be used to localize any clotting or cholesterol crystallization of blood vessels posterior to the eye.[27]

6.6.4 Laboratory Testing

Strokes are commonly diagnosed through physical examinations; however, various laboratory tests are conducted to screen for the potentiality of a stroke. These tests examine the health and function of the brain, vascular system, and the heart.

6.6.5 Computed Tomography

Computed tomography (CT) scan is an imaging test that utilizes radiation to form a cross-sectional image of the brain. An image is able to identify blood vessel abnormalities, malignant growths, as well as blood clots.[29] A CT scan cannot be used to diagnose a stroke, as the brain may not appear abnormal for several hours after the onset of a stroke and may be too minute to be visible. It is, however, conducted to determine if a stroke is of an ischemic or hemorrhagic origin.[29]

6.6.6 Magnetic Resonance Imaging

Magnetic resonance imaging (MRI) scans use magnetic and radio waves to produce a diagnostic image. Similar to CT scans, MRIs are able to detect abnormalities within the brain such as atherosclerotic blood vessels and ultimately detect strokes.[29] MRIs are more accurate compared to CT scans but take considerably more time. MRI scans are not able to accurately identify cytotoxic edema, which is consistent with the acute phase of a stroke. However, it is able to identify vasogenic edema, characteristic of the subacute phase of a stroke.[29]

6.6.7 Carotid Doppler

A carotid Doppler is prescribed to detect atherosclerosis of the carotid artery, where obstruction can result in a stroke.[29] It utilizes ultrasonic technology and is able to detect blood flow through this artery. In comparison to imaging examinations, this test is relatively fast to conduct, and results are immediate.

6.6.8 Electrocardiogram

Electrocardiograms (ECGs) are tests, which monitor the heart's rhythm by using electrodes placed along the body to monitor the electrical activity.[30] It is a broad assessment used to monitor the health of the heart, and is not typically prescribed and cannot be used for the diagnosis of a stroke. However, they are able to diagnose arrhythmias such as atrial fibrillation, a contributing factor for the onset of a stroke.[30]

6.6.9 Other Less Definitive Laboratory Examinations

Other tests may be prescribed for individuals who are at an elevated risk for the development of a stroke. These examinations, however, are unable to diagnose a stroke but will give an indication of the risk factors. Tests include: complete blood count (FBC); blood lipid tests; coagulation test—prothrombin time (PT); homocysteine levels, and blood glucose.[30,31]

6.7 Medical Management and Treatment of Stroke

6.7.1 Secondary Stroke Prevention Post-transient Ischemic Heart Attack

Prescription of warfarin, a vitamin K inhibitor, reduces the incidences of stroke by two-thirds for patients suffering from atrial fibrillation (AF).[32] In addition, the administration of warfarin targeting an international normalized ratio (INR) between 2 and 3 is recommended for AF patients undergoing hemodialysis (HD), decreasing the risk of thromboembolic stroke while maintaining minimal bleeding risk.[32] However, due to a narrow therapeutic index and unpredictable anticoagulation effects, caution should be exercised when warfarin is prescribed to these patients.[32] Antiplatelet therapy can be considered as a possible prophylactic treatment in the case of strokes.[32]

From a preventative perspective, early intervention is paramount as the transient ischemic attack (TIA) and minor stroke patients are at an increased risk for developing recurrent cerebral strokes.[34] Research endorses a combined antiplatelet therapy in conjunction with aspirin as an effective secondary preventative measure for noncardiogenic stroke or TIA.[33,34] The combined therapy is recommended for management, as it is more efficacious when compared to the use of aspirin alone.[33,34] However, discrepancies within the literature show varying outcomes for the same method of prevention. For example, two meta-analyses advocates that a treatment combination of aspirin and Clopidogrel is safe with no increased risk of hemorrhage.[33] In contrast, other studies suggest a combination of aspirin and Clopidogrel as effective in decreasing the risk of recurrent strokes within a 3-month period.[34] However, prolonged use of aspirin and Clopidogrel contributes to major bleeding and hemorrhagic stroke incidents.[34]

6.7.2 Endovascular Treatment for Acute Ischemic Stroke

Acknowledged as one of the leading contributors to global morbidity and mortality rates, an acute ischemic stroke episode can lead to permanent brain tissue damage due to the insufficient perfusion of blood.[35,36] Therefore, intra-arterial mechanical thrombectomy (IMT) in conjunction with intravenous thrombolysis is indicated as it allows the retrieval of clots and effective recanalization.[35,36] Based on the findings of Rodrigues' meta-analysis on endovascular treatment for ischemic stroke, timely intravenous administration of recombinant tissue plasminogen activator (rt-PA) coupled with endovascular interventions significantly improves recanalization rate and reduces the severity of infarction to the brain.[36] Specifically, for patients below the age of 85 experiencing an acute ischemic stroke attack, intravenous thrombolysis is recommended with the administration of rt-PA together with IMT within 6 to 8 hours after onset.[36] Unlike other forms of intervention, this treatment does not pose any risk to mortality or ICH, and conversely, it extends the window of treatment from a standard 4.5 hours to greater than 6 hours.[36] This increases the likelihood of patients being functionally dependent within 3 months post-stroke.[36] Research consistently indicates that the chances of recovery without debilitation is doubled when patients are managed with adjunctive IMT.[36] In addition, meta-analyses have reiterated the success rate and reduction of mortality, when the use of endovascular therapy with or without rt-PA is administered within the 6-hour window post-stroke.[35] It is advocated that a multidisciplinary stroke team is developed in the prevention of stroke, as it allows for a rapid triage and protocol-based approach to achieve optimal clinical outcomes.[35]

6.8 Management of a Dental Patient with Stroke

6.8.1 Special Considerations for Patients on Anticoagulants Undergoing Oral Surgery

As fatal thromboembolic events are more prevalent in elderly patients, they are often prescribed oral anticoagulant therapies (OAT) such as warfarin, heparin, and new oral anticoagulants (NOAC).[37,38] Dental and oral surgical interventions are also prevalent within this population, and thus, it is paramount that postoperative bleeding is kept to a minimum.[37] It is vital that dentists are aware that the discontinuation of OAT in high-risk patients increases the potential for an embolic complication by threefold.[37] An additional meta-analysis has also indicated that the interruption of the course of OAT increases the risk of a lethal thromboembolic incident while making no difference to postoperative bleeding rates.[38] Furthermore, for patients treated with anticoagulants, their INR should be monitored one to two days prior to minor oral surgeries such as dental extractions, to ensure it is within the therapeutic range of 2 to 4 (38–40). An INR of less than 2 increases the risk of thromboembolic events including AF by 50%, while an INR exceeding 5 is associated with the increased incidence of postoperative bleeding.[38] Alternatively, to control the risk of postoperative bleeding, local hemostatic measures such as the use of tranexamic acid mouthwash may be of benefit.[39] Suturing of the wound, however, did not display any therapeutic benefits.[38] Furthermore, for patients treated with OAT undergoing major oral maxillofacial surgery, a bridging therapy of low-molecular-weight heparin is indicated as the preferred treatment.[37] It is of utmost importance that dental practitioners are aware of the potential increase in INR when prescribing nonsteroidal anti-inflammatory drugs to these patients for pain management.[37]

6.8.2 Addressing Oral Hygiene Problems in Post-Stroke Deficits

Stroke is a disease that causes high mortality rates together with morbidity in the form of disability-adjusted life years (DALY).[40] A stroke may cause motor, sensory, and cognitive impairments often resulting in patients experiencing difficulties in maintaining good oral hygiene as their self-care practices are compromised.[41] Therefore, increased dental plaque levels are common in these patients and contribute to oral infections such as dental caries, gingivitis, and periodontitis.[40,41] The bacteria within dental plaque are often opportunistic pathogens, which are also associated with respiratory pneumonia and bacteremia.[40,41] Addressing the increasingly poor oral health within post-stroke patients, a randomized clinical trial evaluated the effectiveness of an advanced oral hygiene care program (AOHCP) and a conventional oral hygiene care program (COHCP).[41] AOHCP details the application of an electrical toothbrush and a mouth rinse containing chlorhexidine, whereas COHCP advises the use of a manual toothbrush only.[41] When comparing both programs, research indicates AOHCP as a more effective regime in the removal of plaque and reduction of gingival bleeding.[41] It is also the program of choice for the integration of oral hygiene care into stroke rehabilitation.[41] Moreover, it is widely acknowledged that due to physical disability, stroke patients experience inequalities in access to dental health services.[40] Despite these inequalities, dentists also express less willingness to treat these patients, as it requires additional considerations and infrastructure.[40]

6.8.3 Prior to and during Dental Treatment

Prior treatment, a thorough patient anamnesis is to be recorded and noted by the clinician. Patients exhibiting a number of the following risk factors: old age, smoking, hypertension, dyslipidemia, cerebrovascular disease, diabetes, and transient vascular accidents, sit highly susceptible to stroke and immediate medical referral is necessary.[42] Dental-specific panoramic radiographs that display carotid calcification in the region of the angle of the mandible also presents as a risk factor for stroke.[42] When accounting for patient's medical history, the practitioner needs also to consider any history of past stroke, myocardial infarction (MI), or TIA as indicators of a possible impending stroke during upcoming treatments.[42] Often preceding a major stroke is several episodes of TIA occurring close together. If the patient experiences these attacks during a treatment session, follow-up phone calls are recommended.

When treating those who present a stroke history, special care, modifications, and considerations should be provided: patients shall be for choice in the morning, appointments shall be short (30–45 minutes), and only operations of minimal stress and pain are to be conducted.[43] Selective premedications may be considered to further benefit patients of this cohort. These include prophylactic nitroglycerine to prevent bacteremia, anxiolytic nitrous oxide-oxygen sedation to minimize anxiety-related heightened blood pressure, and anesthetics administered via slow delivery at a low concentration of epinephrine (1:100,000), if necessary.[44] For those taking warfarin, appropriate laboratory tests for INR values is required and the dose may need to be adjusted accordingly to obtain an ideal INR value of less than 4.0 as described above. If dental treatment risks bleeding, anticoagulant medications should be stopped at least 6 to 12 hours prior, to avoid serious hemorrhage.[45] Medications can be resumed 6 hours post bleeding to allow for sufficient time for blood clot formation.[45] Patients with impaired swallowing should be seated upright, with appropriate use of suctioning and if the patient is in a wheelchair, the practitioner is required to determine the preferred transfer method.[46] Cardiac status and blood pressure should be closely monitored and under control throughout the entire intervention.

Sudden or temporary weakness, numbness of the face, loss of speech, unexplained loss of balance, or dizziness are warning signs of a severe stroke attack and must be recognizable to the clinician.[45] If an apparent stroke has occurred during a dental procedure; provide immediate oxygen therapy, ensure the patient's airways are maintained, and circulation is stable until emergency medical personnel arrive.[47] The patient should be transported to an appropriate medical facility immediately, as definitive management is optimal within 3 hours after onset of symptoms.[47]

For a maximum of 1 year after their stroke or TIA, patients encounter a higher risk of a repeated stroke when compared to their initial attack; 70% of recurrent episodes occur within 1 month.[45] On the basis of this increased risk, it is recommended that dental treatment be delayed for a minimum of 6 months after occurring incidences.[44]

6.9 Oral Medicine Aspects of Stroke

6.9.1 Clinical Diagnosis

The range in orofacial clinical manifestations of stroke is determined by size and location of the affected brain region.[43] The most prevalent signs and symptoms include sensory and motor deficits: facial droop, paresis in extraocular muscles and eye movements, slurred speech, seizures, and neurocognitive deficits.[43] Recognizing these signs and symptoms is the first and most crucial element of stroke care.[47] As a general rule, one has to follow the "Spot a Stroke FAST" protocol (▶ Fig. 6.3). To diagnose a stroke, however, supplementary neurologic and cardiovascular examinations, and anatomic and functional brain imaging, are essential.[43] As discussed in the identification section earlier, brain MRI is the most effective method for localization of stroke sites. Blood counts, urinalysis, and coagulation profile are effective supplementary laboratory evaluation methods for stroke victims.[43]

6.9.2 Nonsurgical Management and Treatment

Subsequent to a stroke attack, patients may experience dysfunctions of the oral region: impairment of touch and taste sensations, diminished protective gag reflex, dysphagia, and aphasia causing alterations in taste satisfaction, chewing capacity, and swallowing.[46] Damage to the facial and trigeminal nerve causes facial and muscle paralysis surrounding the oral cavity. Motor functions of the masticatory and facial muscles will hence be compromised. Consequently, the oral environment's clearance ability will reduce, resulting in food accumulation and packing around teeth and in the folds of the oral mucosa.[46] Aforementioned issues in combination with the possibility of diminished dexterity of arms and hands reduce a patient's oral-health-related quality of life (OHRQoL) and hence overall quality of life.[48] Patients will be at elevated risks of pathological, destructive oral diseases in addition to life-threatening infections including aspiration pneumonia.[49] To rehabilitate and improve OHRQoL, a dental practitioner should consider the following for management and treatment methods.

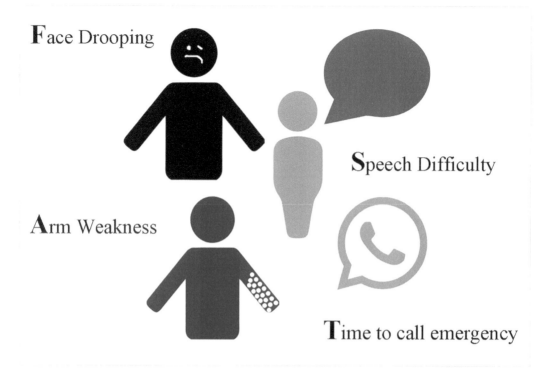

Fig. 6.3 Spot a stroke F.A.S.T.

Frequent Recall Examinations and Dental Prophylaxis

Studies present periodontitis as a correlated risk for stroke. Periodontal infections provide a stable environment for bacterial growth and partake in inflammatory processes that result in the narrowing of blood vessels, increasing stroke risk.[50] In addition, bacteremia of plaque causes increased platelet aggregation involved in embolism, one of the principal causes of stroke.[50]

Provide Oral Hygiene Instructions

As discussed above in the section addressing oral hygiene problems, inform and advise the patient on AOHCP, which comprises the use of electric toothbrushes and 0.2% chlorhexidine mouth rinse.[48] Practitioners may consider pairing oral irrigation instruments with plaque-revealing tablets. This will assist the patient in identifying bacteria-residing areas and necessary areas of focus when brushing and flossing teeth.

Promote Caries Preventative Methods

Due to patient's decreased OHRQoL, their susceptibility to dental caries is heightened; hence, caries preventative methods will be of benefit: prescribe fluoride-containing mouth rinse (e.g., Colgate NeutraFluor, Colgate Dry Mouth Relief), xylitol lozenges (e.g., Xylimelts), and suggest a low cariogenic diet to reduce the burden of caries-promoting bacteria—*Streptococcus mutans*. Advise patients to avoid soft, sticky foods and a diet high in carbohydrates and refined sugars; instead, recommend noncariogenic foods including fresh fruit, vegetables, and savory snacks.

Fixed Prosthodontics Treatment

Edentulous patients or patients with missing teeth are instructed to obtain fixed prosthodontics treatment.[46] This will disregard the difficulties involved with insertion and removal of dentures and aid with chewing and diet.[43]

Antiplatelet and Anticoagulant Medications

Prescribe antiplatelet and anticoagulant medications to treat thromboembolism. Above sections discussed in detail the optimal dosage regimens and their respective roles in the management of stroke. Overall, management of oral health succeeding stroke is integral in preventing and reducing the likelihood of a subsequent stroke, as a result of oral diseases. However, considering no single patient will present identical aftereffects to another, it is essential for practitioners to entirely understand each individual patient's conditions, and construct a personalized treatment plan to optimally accommodate their body's special needs.

6.9.3 Coordination of Care between Dentist and Physician

Primary care physicians and dentists are often the first forms of contact for health care by the public, and hence have a crucial role in the early detection and diagnosis of stroke. Patients who adhere to their dental check-up every 6 months would see their dentists more often than their general practitioners. For many decades, numerous studies have shown a clear association between poor oral health and the onset of systemic diseases. Studies have documented a relationship between periodontitis and progression in noncommunicable diseases such as stroke, coronary heart disease, and arteriosclerosis.[51] Reinforced by the World Health Organization, "oral health is acknowledged as an integral component of overall health and general well-being," but is often overlooked by many other health disciplines in the treatment of chronic diseases.[52]

In a study conducted in Tabriz, Iran to investigate cardiologists' knowledge regarding the "effects of periodontal diseases on coronary heart system," it was found that 76% of cardiologists agreed that control of infection and inflammation is crucial in the management of coronary heart diseases (CHD)[53]; whereby CHD is linked to many other cardiovascular diseases such as stroke and myocardial infarct.

Moreover, most cardiovascular diseases share the same predisposing factors of high cholesterol levels, hypertension, and diabetes. Alongside, 62% of cardiologists reported not having received any oral health care education.[53] Hence, in order to achieve a more comprehensive diagnosis of stroke, it is crucial that general practitioners and dental practitioners cooperate and are appropriately educated in each other's respective field. This will ensure a more effective referral system, so patients are directed to the appropriate professional for necessary treatment.[54]

Dental Treatment of Patients on Anticoagulant Therapy

An example of coordination of care between dentists and physicians is the management of anticoagulant therapy during dental surgery. Dentists play a key role in detecting and referring patients suspected of having ischemic attacks/past stroke episodes or any oral drug reactions, and in partnership with physicians, are responsible for oral and systemic disease prevention and treatment. As mentioned, most stroke patients encountered in the dental clinic will be undertaking anticoagulant or antiplatelet therapy such as Warfarin and aspirin.[55] Due to the potential adverse drug reactions, it is crucial that prior to any dental surgical procedure, close collaboration between dentists and physicians occurs to assess the bleeding risks of continued anticoagulant medication against the risk of post-thrombosis in ceasing anticoagulant medication.[56]

References

[1] Hankey GJ. Stroke. Lancet. 2017; 389(10069):641–654
[2] Cooke M, Cuddy MA, Farr B, Moore PA. Cerebrovascular accident under anesthesia during dental surgery. Anesth Prog. 2014; 61(2):73–77
[3] Hachinski V, Donnan GA, Gorelick PB, et al. Stroke: working toward a prioritized world agenda. Stroke. 2010; 41(6): 1084–1099
[4] Feigin VL, Norrving B, George MG, Foltz JL, Roth GA, Mensah GA. Prevention of stroke: a strategic global imperative. Nat Rev Neurol. 2016; 12(9):501–512
[5] Esenwa C, Gutierrez J. Secondary stroke prevention: challenges and solutions. Vasc Health Risk Manag. 2015; 11:437–450

[6] Al-Shahi R, White PM, Davenport RJ, Lindsay KW. Subarachnoid haemorrhage. BMJ. 2006; 333(7561):235–240

[7] WHO. Global Health Estimates 2015: Deaths by Cause, Age, Sex, by Country and by Region, 2000–2015. World Health Organization; Geneva; 2016

[8] Thomas Truelsen SB. Colin Mathers. Global burden of cerebrovascular disease. WHO Discussion Paper, World Health Organization, Geneva, Switzerland; 2006

[9] Sierra C, Coca A, Schiffrin EL. Vascular mechanisms in the pathogenesis of stroke. Curr Hypertens Rep. 2011; 13(3):200–207

[10] Australian, , Bureau, , Statistics. 2004

[11] Institute of Medicine (US) Committee on Preventing the Global Epidemic of Cardiovascular Disease: Meeting the Challenges in Developing Countries; Fuster V, Kelly BB, editors. Promoting Cardiovascular Health in the Developing World: A Critical Challenge to Achieve Global Health. Washington (DC): National Academies Press (US). Committee on Preventing the Global Epidemic of Cardiovascular Disease: Meeting the Challenges in Developing Countries. https://www.ncbi.nlm.nih.gov/books/NBK45687/. Published 2010. Accessed May 2019

[12] Ovbiagele B, Nguyen-Huynh MN. Stroke epidemiology: advancing our understanding of disease mechanism and therapy. Neurotherapeutics. 2011; 8(3):319–329

[13] Truelsen T, Mähönen M, Tolonen H, Asplund K, Bonita R, Vanuzzo D, WHO MONICA Project. Trends in stroke and coronary heart disease in the WHO MONICA Project. Stroke. 2003; 34(6):1346–1352

[14] WHO. The Atlas of Heart Disease and Stroke. Global Burden of Stroke. 2015

[15] Gubitz G, Sandercock P. Prevention of ischaemic stroke. BMJ. 2000; 321(7274):1455–1459

[16] Rink C, Khanna S. MicroRNA in ischemic stroke etiology and pathology. Physiol Genomics. 2011; 43(10):521–528

[17] Johansson BB. Hypertension mechanisms causing stroke. Clin Exp Pharmacol Physiol. 1999; 26(7):563–565

[18] Hisham NF, Bayraktutan U. Epidemiology, pathophysiology, and treatment of hypertension in ischaemic stroke patients. J Stroke Cerebrovasc Dis. 2013; 22(7):e4–e14

[19] Rubattu S, Giliberti R, Volpe M. Etiology and pathophysiology of stroke as a complex trait. Am J Hypertens. 2000; 13(10):1139–1148

[20] Huang HD, Yang CM, Shu HF, et al. Genetic predisposition of stroke: understanding the evolving landscape through meta-analysis. Int J Clin Exp Med. 2015; 8(1):1315–1323

[21] Markus HS. Stroke genetics. Hum Mol Genet. 2011; 20 R2: R124–R131

[22] Schunkert H, Götz A, Braund P, et al. Cardiogenics Consortium. Repeated replication and a prospective meta-analysis of the association between chromosome 9p21.3 and coronary artery disease. Circulation. 2008; 117(13):1675–1684

[23] Francis J, Raghunathan S, Khanna P. The role of genetics in stroke. Postgrad Med J. 2007; 83(983):590–595

[24] Joutel A, Monet-Leprêtre M, Gosele C, et al. Cerebrovascular dysfunction and microcirculation rarefaction precede white matter lesions in a mouse genetic model of cerebral ischemic small vessel disease. J Clin Invest. 2010; 120(2):433–445

[25] Rutten J, Lesnik Oberstein SAJ. Cadasil. In: Pagon RA, Adam MP, Ardinger HH, Wallace SE, Amemiya A, Bean LJH, et al., eds. GeneReviews(R). Seattle, WA; 1999

[26] Terni E, Giannini N, Brondi M, Montano V, Bonuccelli U, Mancuso M. Genetics of ischaemic stroke in young adults. BBA Clin. 2014; 3:96–106

[27] Torbey MT, Selim MH. The Stroke Book. Cambridge: Glasgow, United Kingdom: Cambridge University Press; 2013.

[28] Wiebers DO, Feigin VL, Brown RD. Handbook of Stroke. 2nd ed. Philadelphia, PA: Lippincott Williams & Wilkins; 2006:480

[29] Markus HS, Pereira A, Cloud G. Stroke Medicine. 2nd ed. Oxford, United Kingdom; New York, NY: Oxford University Press; 2017: xii, 596p

[30] Fisher M, Fisher M. Stroke: Pt. 3: Investigation and Management. Elsevier Imprint; 2008

[31] Gertsch M. The ECG: A Two-Step Approach to Diagnosis. Berlin: Springer; 2004:xxxiv, 615

[32] Li J, Wang L, Hu J, Xu G. Warfarin use and the risks of stroke and bleeding in hemodialysis patients with atrial fibrillation: a systematic review and a meta-analysis. Nutr Metab Cardiovasc Dis. 2015; 25(8):706–713

[33] Zhou X, Tian J, Zhu MZ, He CK. A systematic review and meta-analysis of published randomized controlled trials of combination of clopidogrel and aspirin in transient ischemic attack or minor stroke. Exp Ther Med. 2017; 14(1):324–332

[34] Zhang Q, Wang C, Zheng M, et al. Aspirin plus clopidogrel as secondary prevention after stroke or transient ischemic attack: a systematic review and meta-analysis. Cerebrovasc Dis. 2015; 39(1):13–22

[35] Sardar P, Chatterjee S, Giri J, et al. Endovascular therapy for acute ischaemic stroke: a systematic review and meta-analysis of randomized trials. Eur Heart J. 2015; 36(35):2373–2380

[36] Rodrigues FB, Neves JB, Caldeira D, Ferro JM, Ferreira JJ, Costa J. Endovascular treatment versus medical care alone for ischaemic stroke: systematic review and meta-analysis. BMJ. 2016; 353:i1754

[37] Kämmerer PW, Frerich B, Liese J, Schiegnitz E, Al-Nawas B. Oral surgery during therapy with anticoagulants: a systematic review. Clin Oral Investig. 2015; 19(2):171–180

[38] Yang S, Shi Q, Liu J, Li J, Xu J. Should oral anticoagulant therapy be continued during dental extraction? A meta-analysis. BMC Oral Health. 2016; 16(1):81

[39] Shi Q, Xu J, Zhang T, Zhang B, Liu H. Post-operative bleeding risk in dental surgery for patients on oral anticoagulant therapy: a meta-analysis of observational studies. Front Pharmacol. 2017; 8:58

[40] Dai R, Lam OL, Lo EC, Li LS, Wen Y, McGrath C. A systematic review and meta-analysis of clinical, microbiological, and behavioural aspects of oral health among patients with stroke. J Dent. 2015; 43(2):171–180

[41] Dai R, Lam OLT, Lo ECM, Li LSW, McGrath C. A randomized clinical trial of oral hygiene care programmes during stroke rehabilitation. J Dent. 2017; 61:48–54

[42] Little JW. Dental Management of the Medically Compromised Patient. 8th ed. St. Louis, MO: Elsevier/Mosby; 2013:xii, DM-59, 659

[43] Glick M. Burket's Oral Medicine. 12th ed. Shelton, CT: People's Medical Publishing House; 2015:xv, 716

[44] Ganda KM. Dentist's Guide to Medical Conditions, Medications, and Complications. 2nd ed. Ames, IA: Wiley-Blackwell; 2013:xv

[45] Grotta JC. Stroke: Pathophysiology, Diagnosis, and Management. 6th ed. Philadelphia, PA: Elsevier; 2016:xvi, 1254

[46] Stefanac SJ, Nesbit SP. Diagnosis and Treatment Planning in Dentistry. 3rd ed. St. Louis, MO: Elsevier; 2017:xiv, 445

[47] Lockhart PB. Oral Medicine and Medically Complex Patients. 6th ed. Ames: Wiley-Blackwell; 2013

[48] Dai R, Lam OLT, Lo ECM, Li LSW, McGrath C. Oral health-related quality of life in patients with stroke: a randomized clinical trial of oral hygiene care during outpatient rehabilitation. Sci Rep. 2017; 7(1):7632

[49] Ab Malik N, Mohamad Yatim S, Lam OL, Jin L, McGrath CP. Effectiveness of a Web-Based Health Education Program to

promote oral hygiene care among stroke survivors: randomized controlled trial. J Med Internet Res. 2017; 19(3):e87

[50] Hashemipour MA, Afshar AJ, Borna R, Seddighi B, Motamedi A. Gingivitis and periodontitis as a risk factor for stroke: a case-control study in the Iranian population. Dent Res J (Isfahan). 2013; 10(5):613–619

[51] Sippli K, Rieger MA, Huettig F. GPs' and dentists' experiences and expectations of interprofessional collaboration: findings from a qualitative study in Germany. BMC Health Serv Res. 2017; 17(1):179

[52] Halpern LR, Kaste LM. Impact of Oral Health on Interprofessional Collaborative Practice: An Issue of Dental Clinics of North America. Elsevier Health Sciences; 2016

[53] Atabak Kashefimehr MF, Shirmohammadi A, Zarandi A, Ilkhani S. Awareness regarding the effects of periodontal diseases on coronary heart system among cardiologists in Tabriz, Iran. Periodontology & Implant Dentistry.. 2014; 6(1): 23–27

[54] Smith HA, Smith ML. The role of dentists and primary care physicians in the care of patients with sleep-related breathing disorders. Front Public Health. 2017; 5:137

[55] Chaudhry S, Jaiswal R, Sachdeva S. Dental considerations in cardiovascular patients: a practical perspective. Indian Heart J. 2016; 68(4):572–575

[56] Wahl MJ. Dental surgery and antiplatelet agents: bleed or die. Am J Med. 2014; 127(4):260–267

7 Epilepsy and Other Seizure Disorders

Armin Ariana

Abstract

Epilepsy is a broad umbrella term defining a group of neurological diseases that present with recurrent episodes of seizures. As one of the most prevalent neurological disorders, epilepsy is affecting an estimated 50 million individuals worldwide. Epilepsy is caused by abnormal electrical activity of the brain, which results from uncontrolled discharges and hyperexcitability of groups of neurons. Seizures are characterized by sudden involuntary convulsions, and in some cases, small periods of unawareness that may accompany random, uncharacteristic behaviors in the patient. Epilepsy is a disorder that can present at all ages, affecting both males and females, and commonly caused by genetic predisposition, congenital abnormalities, and antenatal or perinatal injury. The overall objective in management and treatment of epilepsy is complete seizure control for an improved quality of life. Being aware of the health status of a patient diagnosed with epilepsy is critical for health professionals. It is vital that the coordination of care between health professionals' teams exists to ensure the practitioner has all the required information about the patient before initiating any clinical procedures. Appropriate treatment planning and coordination with other health practitioners will ensure the patient's general and dental health is adequately sustained and potential dangers minimized.

Keywords: epilepsy, seizure, epidemiology, pathogenesis, treatment, oral manifestations, medical management

7.1 Background of Epilepsy and Other Seizure Disorders

Epilepsy, one of the most prevalent neurological disorders, is a broad umbrella term that defines a group of diseases that present with recurrent episodes of seizures, affecting an estimated 50 million individuals worldwide. They are regarded as a collection of conditions with different pathophysiologies, multiple manifestations, and diverse etiologies.[1] Seizures are characterized by sudden involuntary convulsions, and in some cases, small periods of unawareness that may accompany random, uncharacteristic behaviors in the patient. While the terms *epilepsy* and *seizures* tend to be used synonymously, they, in fact, describe different but related medical situations. Any healthy brain can be provoked to generate a seizure, be it through drugs, metabolic changes, or trauma. Such self-provoked seizures are not classified as epileptic. Epilepsy is exclusive to seizures that are not self-provoked, and there is an underlying neurological reason for the episodic attacks.[2] Occurrences of repeated seizures lead to the potential diagnosis of epilepsy; however, many other factors must be considered in order for a patient to be diagnosed with epilepsy, including the frequency of unprovoked seizures and risk of recurrence in patients.

7.2 Description of Epilepsy and Other Seizure Disorders

Epilepsy is caused by the abnormal electrical activity of the brain. Specifically, the disease state in the brain results from uncontrolled discharges from groups of neurons—hyperexcitability of the neurons of the cerebral hemispheres.[3] The potential cause of such abnormal brain activity is vast and extensive and may be different for each patient. Some common causes include genetic predisposition, congenital abnormalities, and antenatal or perinatal injury.[3] Epilepsy is a disorder that can present at all ages, affecting both males and females, with males at a slightly higher risk.[3]

Many patients experience warning signs before an impending seizure, such as light-headedness or nausea, usually occurring immediately beforehand. Epileptic attacks can involve several elements alongside the typical uncoordinated twitching of muscles and spastic contractions. Distorted sensory phenomena, altered consciousness, and inappropriate behavior tend to present as well. Postictal (the altered state of conscious after an epileptic seizure) symptoms may comprise headaches, confusion, muscle ache, and drowsiness.[3] This tends to last between 5 and 30 minutes, but sometimes longer in the case of larger, more severe seizures. With such clinical manifestations of epilepsy, many physical and psychosocial consequences may arise. As a result of the lack of consciousness, patients may seriously injure themselves with their behaviors, potentially leading to death. Epileptic patients may also suffer from stigma and as a result educational and vocational impairments, heavily impacting their quality of life.

Seizures, epilepsies, and epilepsy syndromes have been categorized in many forms throughout the years. Classification is of importance, as it is required for correct evaluation and management of patients. Seizures are classified as generalized, simple partial, or complex partial, based on the symptoms observed during the seizure. There are fundamental physiological differences between them, which explain their wide range of clinical manifestations and varied responses to different medications. Generalized seizures involve a loss of consciousness at the onset. The entire cortex is affected concurrently; therefore, cortical neurons that maintain consciousness are unable to function. They are in most cases idiopathic and begin in childhood.[4] Consciousness is retained during partial seizures. Simple partial seizures are localized to a small discrete area of the brain, and the subsequent symptoms are location-dependent, involving only a few muscles on the face, arms, or legs. Seizures arising in the visual cortex of the occipital lobe cause visual abnormalities, while those in the primary motor cortex of the frontal lobe affect hand movements. Complex partial seizures are characterized by an alteration of consciousness, often awake but unresponsive to external stimuli. Automatism, repetitive

purposeless movements, such as lip smacking, hand rubbing, and squeezing, may also manifest.

Treatment of epilepsy involves a number of factors that must be considered. Many antiepileptic drugs (AEDs) exist; however, prescription is based on detailed evaluation of the epileptic patient, which indicates the positive effects of the prescribed drugs will outweigh potential side effects that may manifest. Furthermore, appropriate management of epilepsy extends beyond the prescription of antiepileptic medications; a holistic approach must be adopted—one that addresses social, educational, and psychological issues that the patient may face.

7.3 Epidemiology of Epilepsy

The prevalence of epilepsy is defined as the proportion of those diagnosed with the condition relative to the entire population. The incidence of epilepsy is the rate of diagnosing new cases of the disease within a specified timeframe. The disease is not evenly distributed, appearing more prevalently in developing countries, particularly among individuals of low socioeconomic status, which may be caused by limited access to health treatment, higher incidence of road accident injuries, decreased availability of preventative health measures, and exposure to certain endemic factors such as malaria.[5]

Many studies report the prevalence and incidence of epilepsy to be slightly more pronounced in males, but these differences are statistically insignificant. The prevalence of the disease increases with age in developed countries, while in developing countries it is most prevalent in teenagers and young adults. The incidence is high in infancy and early childhood. Approximately 80% of people with epilepsy in developing countries do not receive appropriate treatment.[5]

Epidemiological differences associated with race are poorly understood, as research comparing ethnic differences within regional populations has not been extensively conducted. The accuracy of epidemiological studies may be inaccurate due to underreporting, as cultural beliefs regarding the causes of the condition lead to heavy stigmatization in certain populations.[5]

7.4 Etiology and Pathogenesis of Epilepsy

Epilepsy is a noncommunicable condition that may be etiologically described as idiopathic, symptomatic, or cryptogenic (▶ Fig. 7.1). Idiopathic forms, which make up approximately 60% of incidences of the disease, have a genetic basis and symptoms manifest early in life. The genetic disorders may be directly related to neuronal dysfunction or may be the result of cortical developmental abnormalities, cavernous and arteriovenous malformations, or neurocutaneous syndrome. The syndrome-specific effects may be the result of a single gene or may follow a complex pattern of inheritance, due to multiple genes and environmental factors.[6]

Symptomatic epilepsies are predominantly acquired following damage to the brain from injuries, tumors, or strokes. Infection of the brain by bacterial, viral, and parasitic organisms may also result in an epileptic disease state, such as in meningitis, encephalitis, or neurocysticercosis. Cryptogenic epilepsies are those to which a cause cannot be readily identified, but which may be eluded upon further investigation.[6]

The incidence of epilepsy is close to 30% in people suffering from brain tumors, whether benign or malignant.[7] The epilepsy risk is dependent on variables such as the presence of cerebral hemispheric dysfunction, hemorrhagic lesions, multiple metastases, and tumor type, grade, or location.[8] A tumor located in the temporal cortex, around the central sulcus or in supplementary areas, is associated with the highest risk for epilepsy development. High-grade malignant tumors grow rapidly and destroy nearby neurons rather than stimulate epileptogenesis; the slow progression of low-grade tumors results in more time for the disease to develop. The comparatively high metabolic rate may lead to hypoxia and interstitial acidosis, which may contribute to disease progression.[5,8,9]

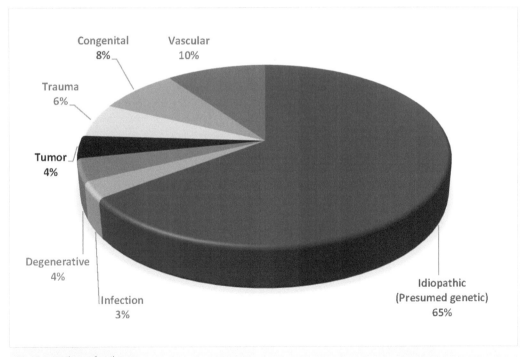

Fig. 7.1 Etiology of epilepsy.

Brain injury has been identified as one of the most vital risk variables for epilepsy development, with up to 20% of epilepsy cases attributed to damage to the brain. The risk of epilepsy is largely dependent on the extent of the injury. Mild brain injuries, characterized by loss of consciousness, amnesia, confusion, and focal temporary neurological deficit, double the epilepsy risk, while a severe brain injury involving intracranial hemorrhage or brain contusion results in a sevenfold higher risk. The risk is highest in the first year following the injury but remains significant even a decade later. The age of the person at the time of the injury is also a factor. Those aged over 15 are more likely to develop epileptic symptoms, as are those with a family history of the disease.[6]

Epilepsy may develop after brain injury as a result of direct cerebral damage or as a consequence of a number of interrelated processes such as edema, ischemia, iron deposition from extravasated blood, or accumulation of glutamate leading to excitotoxicity. Viral meningitis is a common cause of fever-associated seizures. Epilepsy risk is six times higher in those who convulse during meningeal acute illness. Herpes simplex virus is the most common viral epileptogenic agent. The risk is greatest during the first 5 years following infection but remains persistent for 20 years due to the possibility of reactivation of the virus. This may be related to a series of changes such as an increase in proinflammatory cytokines or activation of the immune system.[6,9]

Epilepsy also arises as a consequence of bacterial brain abscesses resulting from head trauma, blood-borne infections, or complications following brain surgery. The risk is greatest in the 3 years following abscess formation. *Streptococcus*, *Staphylococcus*, and gram-negative bacilli are the species typically involved.[6]

7.5 Genetic Component of Seizure Disorders

Although 70 to 80% of cases of epilepsy in the United States have a genetic basis, there is not one uniform genetic disorder responsible for each case of epilepsy.[10,11] Genetic syndromes involved in epilepsy may be the result of copy number variants, deletions of genes, or single-gene mutations.[10,11,12] *SCN1a* and *PCDH19* are two genes that, when mutated, can manifest into a variety of epileptic outcomes that can differ in relation to seizure type, severity, prognosis, and age of onset.[10,11,12,13,14]

SCN1a mutations can lead to the development of a variety of epileptic conditions including generalized epilepsy with febrile seizures plus (GEFS+) and severe myoclonic epilepsy of infancy (SMEI) or Dravet syndrome (DS).[12,14] DS and GEFS+ follow a dominant inheritance pattern or can be de novo mutations.[14] *SCN1a* is a gene on chromosome 2q24 that forms part of a group of nine genes encoding a functional subunit of voltage-gated sodium ion channel 3. Consequently, mutations in the SCN1a group result in a defective sodium ion channel.[12,14] The sodium ion channel is responsible for the depolarization of the plasma membrane when an action potential propagates through a neuron.[14] As the gene can be mutated at any point along its chain, the mutation can be excitatory or inhibitory of central nervous system activity.[14]

Eighty-five percent of SCN1a mutations result in Dravet syndrome. DS is usually the manifestation of a sodium ion channel that has completely lost its function and is associated with intellectual impairment, mental regression, and early onset of seizures.[11,14] Thus, it is a more severe condition when compared to GEFS+ as symptoms other than just seizures are involved. In addition, the degree to which the seizures affect the quality of life of the individual is more severe.[12,14]

Over 50% of the mutations of DS are either frameshift, nonsense, or splice site mutations.[14] Frameshift mutations are the addition or deletion of one or more base pairs during transcription, causing misreading of the genetic code during translation. Nonsense mutations result in a premature stop codon, completely stopping the translation process. Splice site mutations alter where the splicing will occur during translation, resulting in completely different introns and exons and consequently a totally different protein.

Ten percent of SCN1a mutations lead to GEFS + 1, an autosomal-dominant disorder.[10] GEFS + is commonly the outcome of a missense mutation, in which an error of a single nucleotide results in a different amino acid on the mRNA strand. The resulting protein forms a semifunctional sodium channel.[12,14] A defective voltage-gated sodium ion channel may not close once a neuron is depolarized, which leads to hyperexcitable neuronal pathways. Hyperexcitable brain activity can cause spontaneous seizures.[10,12] Seizures may manifest in individuals with GEFS +, but the overall disease is generally less severe than DS as it is not associated with mental disability or refractory seizures.[14]

Protocadherin 19 (*PCDH19*) is a gene on chromosome Xq22.3, which encodes for a transmembrane protein important for neuronal development and the formation of connections between synapses within the brain.[13] During brain development, the transmembrane protein is highly expressed as neuronal pathways are being formed.[13] Mutations in this gene may result in the development of Epilepsy and Mental Retardation Limited to Females (EFMR).

Typically, X-linked inheritance refers to a gene located on the X chromosome. Therefore, males have an increased risk of developing the associated phenotype associated with the gene mutation, as they inherit only a single copy of the mutated allele, unlike females who possess two copies of the X chromosome. This inheritance pattern is commonly seen in color blindness, which affects more males than females. Interestingly, PCDH19 displays X-linked inheritance patterns opposing this standard pattern, and affects only heterozygous females.[13] The disease can be carried through families by asymptomatic male carriers. The reason for this phenomenon is still unknown, but may be the result of a non-paralogous protocadherin gene or other compensatory or rescue factor present on the Y chromosome of males.[13] Epilepsy associated with a PCDH19 mutation is usually associated with intellectual retardation, and brain developmental defects as neuronal development and the formation of synaptic connections are compromised.[13]

7.6 Diagnostic Evaluation of Epilepsy and Seizures

The constitution of what defines epilepsy and seizures involves brain dysfunction, which may manifest as a result of numerous factors. One such definition of an epileptic seizure is "a transient occurrence of signs and symptoms due to abnormal excessive or synchronous neuronal activity in the brain."[15] As it is difficult to identify excessive neuronal activity directly, diagnosis of the seizure-related disease states relies on professional clinical judgment and findings based on medical history, physical examination, and investigation. It is challenging to accurately assess these conditions, as it is not always possible to obtain accurate information regarding the patient's medical history and to ascertain why such a disorder may manifest.[15]

A more practical definition used in a clinical setting sees epilepsy as a disease when two unprovoked seizures are occurring more than 24 hours apart, or one unprovoked seizure and a probability of recurrent seizures over the next 10 years.[15] Understanding of the classification of seizures and epilepsy is crucial for evaluating a patient's medical history during diagnosis (▶ Fig. 7.2).[15] Partial seizures are localized to an area of the brain and may spread. If a patient is conscious, then the diagnosis of a simple partial seizure can be made. Contrary, a generalized seizure does not have a focal onset and awareness by the patient is lost immediately.[16] Generalized seizures are further classed as absence, petit mal, grand mal, myoclonic, atonic, or tonic seizures. It is of importance for a clinician to be aware of conditions that may stimulate seizures, initially addressing if the episode represents a seizure and whether it was provoked.[15]

7.6.1 Medical History

A complete diagnosis of epilepsy is a process that involves discernment of a seizure from other causes of altered consciousness or behavior, differentiation of spontaneous unprovoked seizures from acute symptomatic

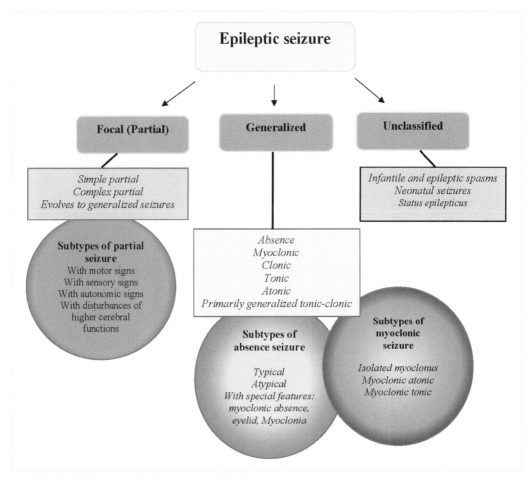

Fig. 7.2 Identification and classification of seizures.

seizures, classification of seizures and epileptic syndromes, and determining the underlying cause.[1] Historical and neurological examinations are the cornerstones of the diagnosis of seizures and epilepsy, while laboratory evaluations serve as adjunctive tests.[17] The context in which an event has occurred must be included when assessing a patient's history. According to Ahmed and Spencer,[16] any witness who can provide additional information regarding the history of the patient should accompany them. The patient should be asked open-ended questions to allow as much detail as possible, and inquiries should center on establishing whether a syndrome is present, guiding the nature of the evaluation, and determining the treatment and prognosis.[17]

Applicable questions include: When did you experience the first seizure in your life? Do you experience some kind of a warning or unusual feeling at the onset, or immediately preceding the seizure? What happens during the seizure? What happens immediately after the seizure? Is there a diurnal variation? Are there any known triggering factors? What is the seizure frequency? What has been the maximum seizure-free period since the seizure onset? Is there more than one kind of seizure? Have the patient sustained injuries related to the seizures? What is the frequency of visits to the emergency department? Is the patient using medications for daily or conditional use?[16]

Details of the patient's birth such as labor and delivery, age-appropriate developmental

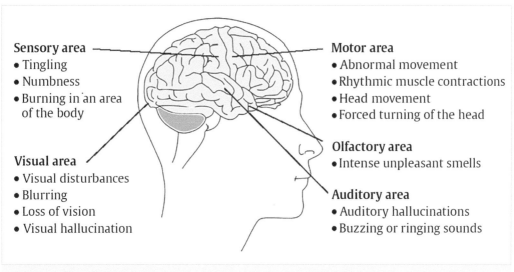

Sensory area
- Tingling
- Numbness
- Burning in an area of the body

Visual area
- Visual disturbances
- Blurring
- Loss of vision
- Visual hallucination

Motor area
- Abnormal movement
- Rhythmic muscle contractions
- Head movement
- Forced turning of the head

Olfactory area
- Intense unpleasant smells

Auditory area
- Auditory hallucinations
- Buzzing or ringing sounds

Fig. 7.3 Symptoms of a localized seizure.

milestones, history of febrile seizures, central nervous system infections, head injuries, brain tumors, or cerebrovascular accidents are considered to be relevant medical history information that provides a useful guide in the classification of the type of epilepsy. Allergies and familial history are also important to determine specific syndromes or other genetically mediated neurological disorders.[16]

Misdiagnosis often occurs when epilepsy in adults is mistaken for syncope or nonepileptic attacks. One of the most common reasons for misdiagnosis is inadequate history taking, and not obtaining an accurate statement from eye-witnesses who were present as the medical situations unfolded.[1]

Physical Examination

A general physical examination is important to determine whether the patient has any underlying pathologies. This should be used to uncover evidence of past or recent head traumas, infections of the ears or sinuses, congenital abnormalities, neurological abnormalities, indications of alcohol or drug abuse, and signs of malignancy.[18] Although seldom possible, observation of a patient during a seizure can provide invaluable information regarding the nature of the patient's distinct condition. Observations of closed eyes during a seizure, resisted eye opening, gaze avoidance, retained pupillary light reflex, semi-purposeful movements, responsiveness to corneal reflex, normal plantar responses would support the diagnosis of nonepileptic seizures. Conversely, patients who experience generalized tonic–clonic seizures often show lateral tongue biting, bruising, skeletal injury, and hemorrhages of the skin or conjunctiva.[19] Observations and findings of facial asymmetry, asymmetry of the thumb size, drift or outstretched hand, dystonic posture when walking, or naming difficulty may expose focal brain dysfunction indicative of symptomatic focal epilepsy (▶ Fig. 7.3).[18]

7.6.2 Laboratory Testing

In almost every case of a first seizure, investigations are initially directed at identifying the precipitating etiology and conditions that can be arrested, reversed, or treated. This information is chiefly resolved through physical examinations and typically followed up using laboratory tests.[16] Predominantly, the two most important predictors of seizures are the presence of abnormalities on an electroencephalogram (EEG) and an underlying neurological disorder that manifests in neurological examinations or neuroimaging.[15] Neurological examinations assess focal signs that might implicate or localize cerebral pathology.[17]

7.6.3 Blood Tests

Routine laboratory investigations such as those that measure serum electrolytes, calcium, magnesium, and toxicology analyses are customarily employed to identify acute provoking factors present in the progression of epilepsy.[15] Curiously, serum prolactin levels have been demonstrated to upsurge as a repercussion of an epileptic seizure.[20] Prolactin is the hormone that is released from the pituitary gland as a result of the propagation of epileptic activity from the temporal lobe to the hypothalamic–pituitary axis. The intensity of the discharge sees a rise in prolactin levels in approximately 78% of patients with complex partial seizures. Postictal serum levels, however, are reportedly more important when differentiating between epileptic and nonepileptic attacks such as syncope and should be measured 30 minutes after the event.[20] Although this serves as a useful method of differentiation, prolactin levels do not confirm an epileptic seizure has occurred and should only be used when EEG is not available.

7.6.4 Neuroimaging

The role of neuroimaging is to detect underlying cerebral abnormalities that may be related to epilepsy or impairments.[21] Computed tomography (CT) or magnetic resonance imaging (MRI) should be considered in any patient who presents with their first seizure as an adjunct to clinical examinations and EEG. While CT is of value in an acute emergency setting to detect hemorrhage, calcification, or tumors, MRI is more likely to show abnormality in patients with focal seizures, abnormal neurological findings, or discharges on EEG due to its improved sensitivity and resolution, making it the more preferred method of detection.[17] Due to the ability of MRI to detect small structural and subtle lesions, it remains an essential part of the presurgical investigation and is the imaging modality of choice when investigating radiological structures in patients.[1] In a series of adults with chronic epilepsy, MRI facilitated findings of the cause in more than 50% of cases, in contrast to CT that enabled 9 to 17% of findings in adults.[21] The ability to image early in epilepsy aids the detection of cases that may require urgent attention, such as tumors, acute stroke or hemorrhage, encephalitis, leukodystrophy, hydrocephalus, or other findings which suggest metabolic or neurogenetic disorders.[21]

More recently, the use of functional MRI (fMRI) is becoming prevalent and may replace traditional single-photon emission computed tomography (SPECT) and positron emission tomography (PET) imaging. It is a noninvasive technique that locates eloquent brain functions such as language-processing areas, which can be spared during resection of the brain.[21]

7.7 Medical Management and Treatment of Epilepsy

The management and treatment of epilepsy take place in several steps with the overall objective being complete seizure control for an improved quality of life. First, the disease must be classified and diagnosed for the particular individual, as certain AEDs are more effective for specific forms of the disease. Understanding the patient's priorities, wants, and needs will also assist in choosing the best drug with side effects that will not impact life issues important to the patient.[22] Approximately half of AED users will achieve seizure control either through long-term monotherapy (the use of a single AED) or polytherapy (two or more AEDs). If the patient relapses despite polytherapy, this indicates pharmacoresistance and the need for other treatment methods.[23] The following are the major AEDs commonly used to treat epilepsy and seizure disorders[24,25]:

Epileptic drugs block the calcium and sodium channels in the membranes of motor neurons, which depresses the spread of an action potential by increasing the threshold needed to initiate a signal.[25] Hence, the occurrence of seizures is decreased. Consequently, this is why many antiseizure drugs cause lethargy.

When first administering epileptic medication, it is better to start off with a lower dose or reduced frequency in order to minimize the adverse effects that are most commonly felt at the beginning of therapy.

Surgical removal of the epileptogenic mass is the next viable solution. The probability of success must be calculated for the patient and depends on the location of the focus tissue. If the process inflicts another neurological problem, then it cannot be considered successful.[23]

If surgical treatment is not an option or was unsuccessful, neuromodulation is the least-preferred treatment method due to its somewhat ineffective 5 to 10% chance of effectual seizure regulation. Vagal nerve stimulation (VNS) is the most traditional and established technique; however, its mechanisms of action are still not understood absolutely. An electrode is implanted in the left cervical area coiling around the Vagus nerve. The electrode is stimulated at regular intervals, which has been observed as having a positive effect in relation to the frequency of seizure episodes. Moreover, the electrode can be manually stimulated in situations where the patient senses the onset of a seizure.[23]

7.8 Management of a Dental Patient with Seizure Disorder

7.8.1 Management of Patient before Dental Treatment

As a dentist expecting to see an epileptic or seizure-prone patient, it is important to take precautions both prior to and during treatment to minimize the risk of seizure and other related health complications. There is an emphasis on preventing causative factors for seizures, often related to stress while in the dental clinic, and customizing treatments to best suit the patient's specific needs.

Before beginning any treatment, the patient's neurologist and pediatrician (if applicable) should be consulted to ensure the safety of such procedures.[26] Although the majority of patients with seizure disorders are likely to be diagnosed already, dentists should still remain wary of signs that may indicate a patient could be suffering from seizures. These signs could include unusual changes in personality, difficulty carrying out normal tasks, or memory issues.[27] For known risk patients, it is essential to minimize stress and anxiety as these often are the underlying causes of seizures. Factors that may trigger stress include loud noises from dental apparatus, bright operating lights,[26] long procedures without sufficient breaks, toothaches, and other painful dental complications.[28] To reduce these possible causative factors, care should be taken to book appointments at a time best suited to the patient, i.e., when they are least susceptible to seizures.[26] It is recommended that dental appointments are scheduled in the morning, as it will minimize the stress and anxiety of the patient, before and during the procedure. Appointments should be kept as short as possible and any sources of pain tended to immediately.[28]

Demonstrating and explaining procedures prior to performing them will also aid in decreasing anxiety, and the dentist, themselves, should exhibit calmness and patience to help keep the patient at ease.[27] Lights are another factor that can trigger an epileptic seizure.[29] Therefore, it is best that the patient wears dark-shaded safety glasses to filter the operating lights.[26]

People with epilepsy or seizure disorders tend to have poorer oral hygiene due to the difficulties encountered during dental visits. Consequently, it is essential that these patients are given thorough oral health instruction (OHI), advising on implementing fluoride products in their daily care and avoid consuming cariogenic foods on a frequent basis.[28] OHI may include a focus on preventative products including electric toothbrushes, proxabrushes for cleaning between teeth, fluoride toothpaste, mouthrinses, etc. A specialized toothbrush such as the Collis-Curve brush may prove beneficial for the patient since its design allows the occlusal, lingual, and facial surfaces of the teeth to be cleaned simultaneously—enabling a more efficient and simpler method of brushing as opposed to regular toothbrushes.[28]

Prescribed AEDs must also be taken before treatment begins.[26] Knowing which AEDs the patient is taking is important since medications prescribed by the dentist often interact with these drugs, reducing their effectiveness and putting the patient at risk. Also, oral side effects of these drugs should be known and tended to by the dentist (▶ Table 7.1). The following briefly describes the relevance of common AEDs:

- Phenytoin: due to gingival hyperplasia, the patient should be recalled more often than regular for removing hyper-plastic tissue through gingivectomy, associated calculus, and preventing plaque formation.
- Carbamazepine: may cause side effects such as ulcers,[27] microbial infections, delayed healing, excessive bleeding,[26] and stomatitis.[28] It is critical to take these effects into consideration before planning any type of invasive procedure and ensure approval with patient's doctor is sought out first. However, approval is generally not necessary for minor operations such as tooth removal.[28] Avoid the use of other medications metabolized by the liver, as their bioavailability will be reduced.
- Phenobarbital: ensure patient stays awake in the chair; it is known to reduce the duration and action of many lipid- and non–lipid-soluble drugs, so avoid drugs that are metabolized in the liver.
- Primidone: should have frequent checking of the density of bone on radiographs.
- Osteoporosis changes facial bone structure: meaning more denture adjustments of removable prosthetics.[4]
- Valproic acid: antibiotics may be prescribed after invasive procedures to avoid/treat infection; reduced dose of analgesics must be given due to enhanced effects.
- Lamotrigine: may need assistance sitting and leaving the dental chair.
- Topiramate: confirm taste sensation changes before injection of local anesthetic.[4]

7.9 Management of Patient during Dental Treatment

Aside from facilitating a stress-free environment and implementing precautionary actions to avoid spurring onset of a seizure, it is important to also understand which materials and treatment options may be best suited to an epileptic patient.

When dealing with prostheses, each case must be considered individually and the best

Table 7.1 Antiepileptic drugs and their oral side effects

Generic name	Brand name	Side effects
Phenytoin sodium	Dilantin	When taken over long periods of time as a chronic drug it can cause gingival hyperplasia or overgrowth, fatigue, skin inflammation, eczema
Carbamazepine	Tegretol	Reduced number of platelets (thrombocytopenia) and white blood cells (leukopenia) in the blood, increased chance of patient's bleeding, infection, and healing retardation, vertigo, light-headedness, nausea, rash, cloudy vision, double vision (diplopia), hepatic enzyme inducer
Phenobarbital	Luminal	Sedation, hypnosis, anemia
Primidone	Mysoline	Osteoporosis and loss of bone density, reduced central nervous system activity, folic acid deficiency
Clonazepam	Klonopin	Increased salivary flow, tachycardia, shakiness, lethargy, frailty,
Valproic acid	Depakene	Has antiplatelet effects, which may cause excessive bleeding due to thrombocytopenia, irritable bowels, e.g., bloating, constipation, diarrhea, weight loss
Lamotrigine	Lamictal	Loss of coordination and voluntary control of muscles (ataxia), dizziness, vomiting, diplopia (double vision)
Topiramate	Topamax	Osteoporosis and loss of bone density. Changes in taste sensation, mood swings, core temperature elevation, fatigue

option for the patient's situation chosen. Normally, however, removable partial dentures are avoided, and fixed appliances are favored due to reduced risk of the appliance dislodging and obstructing the patient's airway.[28] With all factors considered, if a removable denture is still deemed advantageous, a metal base is usually preferred because of its strength and resistance to breakage.[26] Often, issues arise regarding prosthesis retention as a result of developmental changes in the patient. The patient or patient's carer should thus be informed of this risk and that a more stable solution can be reached after jaw growth ceases.[26]

As per usual moisture control practices, rubber dams should always be used unless there is a significant observable risk to the patient's safety.[28] For larger restorative procedures, bridges and metal crowns tend to have better longevity and are less susceptible to breakage during seizures, in comparison to amalgam.[28]

In regard to anesthetics, there is a debate about the safety of its usage with epileptic patients. Sedatives such as nitrous oxide are generally considered safe and suitable for seizure-prone patients. General anesthesia is also considered suitable; however, it may not be the most practical method when performing relatively short and simple procedures—also, it poses a risk of oxygen deprivation (hypoxia) to the brain.[26,28] Local anesthetic, which is the preferred choice for regular dental procedures, is reported to cause problems for people with epilepsy, especially in the case of an overdose as it interacts with AEDs, putting the patient at risk of tonic–clonic convulsions. However, if given in a low dosage, local anesthesia can be fairly safe and effective.[28]

A dentist should always be prepared in the event that a seizure does occur despite implementing precautions as directed. If a seizure occurs, surrounding equipment must be moved away, the chair lowered into the supine position, any materials in the mouth removed and the head turned sideways to open up the airways.[27] Following a seizure, the patient may become unconscious or fall asleep, so it is imperative to ensure their airways remain

unobstructed. Drugs may be necessary if the seizure extends beyond a few minutes and occurs again. If the seizure continues, emergency services must be contacted immediately and the dental appointment deferred for a later date.[27,28]

7.10 Oral Medicine Aspects of Seizure Disorders

Contemporary dentistry utilizes local anesthetics, vasoconstrictors, antibiotics, and pain relief medications. If a patient has been diagnosed with epilepsy or a seizure disorder or is currently taking medication, the effects of the drugs used in the treatment of the individual's dental issues must be considered about how it may affect the overall well-being of the individual.

7.10.1 Local Anesthetic

The local anesthetics typically employed in dentistry comprise of an aromatic ring, an amide linkage (historically an ester linkage), a hydrocarbon chain, and a tertiary amine group.[30] Ester-linked local anesthetics are no longer used due to the bodies breakdown of the ester linkage into *para*-aminobenzoic acid which is the common cause of allergic reactions.[31] Amide-linked local anesthetics are metabolized in the body to inactive metabolites, and true allergic reactions to this group of drugs is rare.[30] Lignocaine is the most widely used dental local anesthetic and therapeutic guidelines limit dosage to 7 mg/kg in the presence of a vasoconstrictor and 3 mg/kg without a vasoconstrictor.[30,31]

Phenytoin is a common AED prescribed to manage epilepsy.[31,32] If present within normal maintained levels, it is not of great concern to the dentist, yet it should be kept in mind that lignocaine and phenytoin have additive effects on the cardiac electrical system and at high doses may lead to sinoatrial arrest.[30,33] The presence of phenytoin may also increase the likelihood of a lignocaine-induced seizure; however, this chance is only elevated at high doses for both drugs.[30,34]

7.10.2 Vasoconstrictors

The use of vasoconstrictors in conjunction with local anesthetics allows the dentist more working time (enhanced analgesic effect) without increasing the dose of local anesthetic due to the vasoconstrictor constraining the local anesthetic to a smaller area.[30] Epinephrine is a catecholamine vasoconstrictor and is widely used; however, when patients are medicated with adrenergic blockers, some dentists prefer to use Felypressin, a non-catecholamine vasoconstrictor.[30]

Epinephrine has been known to induce arrhythmias in patients at doses of 1 mg/kg, particularly those patients under halothane anesthesia.[31,35] Dental procedures are generally not performed under halothane anesthesia and do not utilize epinephrine in comparable doses. The common dose of epinephrine per local anesthetic cartridge being 27.5 mcg or 1:80,000[31] and to reach 1 mg epinephrine, a dentist would need to administer 37 cartridges which would generally exceed the maximum amount of lignocaine permitted under the Australian regulatory guidelines. In any case, it was found that patients taking phenytoin for epilepsy had a better resistance to developing an arrhythmia even in the presence of epinephrine.[30,31]

It should also be noted that many AEDs (such as primidone, lamotrigine, topiramate, and others) amplify drowsiness and impair alertness, while the injections administered during dental treatment, typically containing local anesthetic and a vasoconstrictor, produce an opposing stimulatory effect.[30,31] Although it is not of major concern, the patient's alertness should always be monitored discretely while dental procedures are taking place.

7.10.3 Pain Relief

The advice given by dentists on pain relief is largely regarding over-the-counter medications such as ibuprofen and paracetamol. Carbamazepine administered on a regular basis to manage epilepsy can decrease the effectiveness of ibuprofen due to altering the pathway of metabolism within the body.[22,27,30,31] A better course of action for these patients is paracetamol as the pain relief will be unimpeded and more effective.

Ibuprofen affects the body's metabolic pathways for primidone, phenobarbital, and valproic acid. The effects of primidone will be decreased while the effects of phenobarbital and valproic acid will be increased; both of these outcomes are undesirable and should be avoided.[22,31] The dentist should opt for other options such as paracetamol in order to avoid issues with the patient's epilepsy status.

7.10.4 Antibiotics

Amoxicillin and erythromycin are widely used in Australia and are specifically prescribed by dentists for infections in the oral cavity. The major issue, particularly with erythromycin, is that it may increase the plasma concentration of carbamazepine due to its effect on the body.[36] This leaves the epileptic patient open to the side effects of high doses of carbamazepine and should be discussed with the patient's general practitioner before commencing the prescription.[36]

7.11 Coordination of Care between Dentist and Physician

Being aware of the health status of a patient diagnosed with epilepsy is critical for dental health professionals. It is vital that the coordination of care between dental professionals and physicians is existent to ensure the dentist has all the required information about the patient before initiating any clinical procedures. Communication between the patient's dentist and physician is crucial to ensure the individual's situation is comprehended.[37] The specific details that should be disclosed include the patient's classification of epilepsy, the type of medication they are on, consolidation of their medical history, details on any specific trigger that may result in seizure, and precautions that may need to be taken into account prior to performing a major dental procedure.

When a dental practitioner obtains a medical health history from an epileptic patient, it is of importance that the practitioner consults with the patient's physician to consolidate the results. This is crucial to ensure that the patient's medical history is up to date and the details of their type of epilepsy are known. Knowing the details of the individual's epilepsy case ensures the safest environment for not only the patient but the dental practitioner also.

Obtaining medication information from an epileptic patient's physician is important for a dental practitioner. "Approximately 80% of epilepsy patients are on controlled medication."[38] AEDs are used to treat and prevent seizures and can cause many adverse side effects. Some of these effects include xerostomia, stomatitis, gingivitis, glossitis, oral facial edema, dyspepsia, and gingival hyperplasia.[38] Other adverse effects of AEDs that dental practitioners need to be aware of is dizziness, drowsiness, gastrointestinal upset, and ataxia.[29] It is known that anticonvulsants can cause pathological changes in the oral cavity also. Some signs of changes include irritation and soreness of tongue and mouth, bleeding gums, and swelling of the face, lips, and tongue. Communication between dental practitioners and physicians about an epileptic patient's medical information is important as it allows dental practitioners to be aware of what side effects they could expect to see and also how clinical procedures may interact with the patient's type of medication.

It has been recommended that if a major dental procedure is planned for an epileptic patient, the patient should consult their physician to identify any particular risks and precautions they should prepare for.[29] Knowing the detailed precautions behind a patient's case allows for the dentist to be prepared and knowledgeable. This knowledge to the dentist obtained via communication with the physician will allow for the best possible, structured, and planned procedure and thereby obtain the best procedural outcome.

Epilepsy and related seizure disorders continue to be the major neurological disease affecting people worldwide. The conditions are caused by abnormal excessive neuronal activity in the brain that causes episodes of uncontrolled movement and associated symptoms such as loss of awareness or consciousness. The cause of the illnesses may be due to genetic factors or due to injury to the brain as a result of trauma or pathogen infestation. Disorders are diagnosed through analysis of medical histories, physical exams, and neuroimaging. Treatment may be pharmacological via AEDs, or surgical intervention may be required. Instances of these diseases are especially prevalent in developing countries due to the restricted availability of appropriate health care and medications, higher prevalence of infectious diseases and traumatic accidents, and in some communities, stigmatization associated with the manifestation of the disease.

Although particular requirements and precautions must be satisfied to deliver safe and effective dental treatment of epileptic patients, a knowledgeable and aware clinician can safely manage these cases in an unspecialized dental clinic. An understanding of the patient's medical history and current medications is paramount to providing effectual nonhazardous oral treatment care. Appropriate treatment planning, as well as coordination with the physician, will ensure the patient's oral and general health is adequately sustained and potential dangers minimized.

References

[1] Appleton R, Nicolson A, Chadwick D, MacKenzie J, Smith D. Atlas of Epilepsy. CRC Press; 2006

[2] Wiebe S. The Epilepsies. Goldman's Cecil Medicine. Elsevier; 2012: 2283–2294

[3] Knake S, Hamer HM, Rosenow F. Status epilepticus: a critical review. Epilepsy Behav. 2009; 15(1):10–14

[4] Ganda KM. Dentist's Guide to Medical Conditions, Medications, and Complications. John Wiley & Sons, Ltd; 2013

[5] Bhalla D, Godet B, Druet-Cabanac M, Preux P-M. Etiologies of epilepsy: a comprehensive review. Expert Rev Neurother. 2011; 11(6):861–876

[6] Shneker BF, Fountain NB. Epilepsy. Dis Mon. 2003; 49(7): 426–478

[7] Liigant A, Haldre S, Õun A, et al. Seizure disorders in patients with brain tumors. Eur Neurol. 2001; 45(1):46–51

[8] Banerjee PN, Filippi D, Allen Hauser W. The descriptive epidemiology of epilepsy: a review. Epilepsy Res. 2009; 85(1): 31–45

[9] Thomas RH, Berkovic SF. The hidden genetics of epilepsy: a clinically important new paradigm. Nat Rev Neurol. 2014; 10 (5):283–292

[10] Kullmann DM. Genetics of epilepsy. J Neurol Neurosurg Psychiatry. 2002; 73 Suppl 2:II32–II35

[11] Myers CT, Mefford HC. Advancing epilepsy genetics in the genomic era. Genome Med. 2015; 7(1):91

[12] Mulley JC, Scheffer IE, Petrou S, Dibbens LM, Berkovic SF, Harkin LA. SCN1A mutations and epilepsy. Hum Mutat. 2005; 25(6):535–542

[13] Depienne C, LeGuern E. PCDH19-related infantile epileptic encephalopathy: an unusual X-linked inheritance disorder. Hum Mutat. 2012; 33(4):627–634

[14] Escayg A, Goldin AL. Sodium channel SCN1A and epilepsy: mutations and mechanisms. Epilepsia. 2010; 51(9):1650–1658

[15] Gilliam F. Diagnosis and Classification of Seizures and Epilepsy. Youmans Neurological Surgery. Elsevier; 2011:672–677

[16] Ahmed SN, Spencer SS. An approach to the evaluation of a patient for seizures and epilepsy. WMJ. 2004; 103(1):49–55

[17] Stafstrom CE, Carmant L. Seizures and epilepsy: an overview for neuroscientists. Cold Spring Harb Perspect Med. 2015; 5(6):a022426

[18] Browne TR, Holmes GL. Epilepsy. N Engl J Med. 2001; 344(15):1145–1151

[19] Sirven JI. Diagnosing and Localizing Seizures at the Bedside and in Clinic. Epilepsy. John Wiley & Sons; 2014:33–41

[20] Bauer J. Epilepsy and prolactin in adults: a clinical review. Epilepsy Res. 1996; 24(1):1–7

[21] Novotny EJ. What Can Neuroimaging Tell Us? Epilepsy. John Wiley & Sons; 2014:54–60

[22] Chong DJ. The medical management of epilepsy. Panminerva Med. 2011; 53(4):217–226

[23] Gschwind M, Seeck M. Modern management of seizures and epilepsy. Swiss Med Wkly. 2016; 146:w14310

[24] Henry RG. Neurological Disorders: The ADA Practical Guide to Patients with Medical Conditions. John Wiley & Sons, Inc.; 2015:299–324

[25] Little JW, Falace DA, Miller CS, Rhodus NL. Neurologic, behavioral, and psychiatric disorders. Little and Falace's Dental Management of the Medically Compromised Patient. 9th ed. Elsevier; 2017:716

[26] Joshi SR, Pendyala GS, Saraf V, Choudhari S, Mopagar V. A comprehensive oral and dental management of an epileptic and intellectually deteriorated adolescent. Dent Res J (Isfahan). 2013; 10(4):562–567

[27] Patton LL, Glick M. The ADA Practical Guide to Patients with Medical Conditions. John Wiley & Sons, Inc.; 2015

[28] Mehmet Y, Senem Ö, Sülün T, Hümeyra K. Management of epileptic patients in dentistry. Surg Sci. 2012; 03(01):47–52

[29] Vivek R. Epileptic patients in dentistry: a challenge. J Med Sci Clin Res 2016; 4(4):10154–10157

[30] Rang HP, Dale MM, Ritter JM, Flower RJ. Local anaesthetics and other drugs affecting sodium channels Rang & Dale's Pharmacology. 8th ed. Elsevier; 2016:530–533

[31] Frankhuijzen AL. Pharmacology of Local Anaesthetics. Local Anaesthesia in Dentistry. Springer International Publishing; 2017:37–50

[32] Temkin NR, Dikmen SS, Wilensky AJ, Keihm J, Chabal S, Winn HR. A randomized, double-blind study of phenytoin for the prevention of post-traumatic seizures. N Engl J Med. 1990; 323(8):497–502

[33] Wood RA. Sinoatrial arrest: an interaction between phenytoin and lignocaine. BMJ. 1971; 1(5750):645

[34] Stone WE, Javid MJ. Anticonvulsive and convulsive effects of lidocaine: comparison with those of phenytoin, and implications for mechanism of action concepts. Neurol Res. 1988; 10(3):161–168

[35] Mammoto T, Kamibayashi T, Hayashi Y, Yamatodani A, Takada K, Yoshiya I. Antiarrhythmic action of rilmenidine on adrenaline-induced arrhythmia via central imidazoline receptors in halothane-anaesthetized dogs. Br J Pharmacol. 1996; 117(8):1744–1748

[36] Carranco E, Kareus J, Co S, Peak V, Al-Rajeh S. Carbamazepine toxicity induced by concurrent erythromycin therapy. Arch Neurol. 1985; 42(2):187–188

[37] Ha JF, Longnecker N. Doctor-patient communication: a review. Ochsner J. 2010; 10(1):38–43

[38] Schramke CJ, Kay KA, Valeriano JP, Kelly KM. Using patient history to distinguish between patients with non-epileptic and patients with epileptic events. Epilepsy Behav. 2010; 19(3):478–482

8 Myasthenia Gravis

Armin Ariana

Abstract

Myasthenia gravis is an autoimmune neuromuscular disorder hallmarked by fatigability and weakness of all striated muscles. The clinical features arise from antibodies attacking receptors of the neuromuscular junction, causing impairment of communication between nerves and muscles leading to the generalized or localized weakness and fatigue. The clinical features of the disease, impacts and selection of medications, and modality of treatment are key factors with which clinicians should be thoroughly familiar. Muscles that are often involved in the disease are those that regulate facial expression, talking, eye and limb movement, chewing, and swallowing. The nature of the disease presents challenges to health practitioners and especially dentists in dental management of those diagnosed with myasthenia gravis. The manifestations of myasthenia gravis influence dental treatment, with patients requiring special management considerations to ensure safe and optimal dental treatment. Involvement of facial muscles and muscles of mastication requires careful treatment planning in order to prevent overactivity of the muscles, and exacerbation of the fatigability and weakness that hallmarks this disorder while the patient is undergoing a dental treatment.

Keywords: myasthenia gravis, epidemiology, pathogenesis, treatment, oral manifestations, medical management

8.1 Background of Myasthenia Gravis

Myasthenia gravis (MG) is an autoimmune disorder of the neuromuscular junction (NMJ) hallmarked by fatigability and weakness of all striated muscles. An oral health care provider is likely to encounter more than one patient with this disease throughout their career as approximately 1 in 10,000 people carry the condition.[1] The manifestations of MG influence dental treatment, with patients requiring special management considerations to ensure safe and optimal dental treatment. The clinical features of the disease, impacts and selection of medications, and modality of treatment are key factors with which dentists should be thoroughly familiar. Recent research on MG and approaches to treatment and management of patients in the oral health setting are presented in this chapter.

8.2 Description of Myasthenia Gravis

Myasthenia gravis is an autoimmune neuromuscular disorder marked by fluctuating degrees of weakness of the voluntary (skeletal) muscles of the body, with deterioration during periods of action and improvement following periods of rest.[2] MG was first clinically recognized by neuroanatomist, Thomas Willis, in 1672.[3] The clinical features arise from antibodies attacking receptors of the NMJ, causing impairment of communication between nerves and muscles leading to the generalized or localized weakness and fatigue.[3] Muscles that are often involved in the disease are those that regulate facial expression, talking, eye and limb movement, chewing, and swallowing.[2] In some instances, the involvement of respiratory and bulbar muscles can be life-threatening.[4] These manifestations adversely affect the quality of life, with the patients experiencing difficulty walking a long distance, rising from sitting position, loss of employment, and impairment of carrying out adequate oral hygiene and ability to wear dentures.[1]

The nature of the disease presents challenges to oral health workers in dental management of those diagnosed with MG. Involvement of masticatory and facial muscles requires careful treatment planning in order to prevent overactivity of the muscles.[5] In addition, exacerbation of the fatigability and weakness that hallmarks this disorder can potentially be precipitated by certain medications used by a dentist, signifying that MG patients have specific requirements while undergoing dental treatment.[3] Here we review the epidemiology, etiology, pathogenesis, clinical features, diagnosis, and medical management of MG, and discuss the role of a dentist, in coordination with a physician, in providing oral care and managing the dental complications that may arise from the disorder.

8.3 Epidemiology of Myasthenia Gravis

Epidemiology is the study of patterns, causes, and effects of the disease in a population. It helps identify risk factors for the disease, in this case, MG, and assists in providing preventive solutions. The main feature is the measurement of disease outcome in a population at risk. MG is quite an uncommon disease; however, prevalence has increased in recent times.[6] The National Epidemiological study of MG in Australia (2012) reported an incidence rate of 24.9 per one million residents. Prevalence rates of 117.1 per million residents were found overall. The crude incidence in women was 21.9 per million and men was 27.9 per million. The incidence and prevalence rates were lower in men than women between the ages of 15 and 64 years. However, the prevalence and incidence rates were lower in women over the age of 65. Symptoms can occur from as young as 2 years of age, with the mean age of onset being 43.4 years for women and 53.4 years for men. It was also found that MG disproportionately affected younger females and older males.[7] In a systematic review, it was found that the most accurate estimate of the incidence of MG was around 30 per million a year and the incidence in children and adolescents was between 1 and 5 per million per year.[8] This is similar to the results discussed previously from the National Epidemiological study in Australia by Gattellari.[7]

8.3.1 Distribution of Myasthenia Gravis

The occurrence of MG is influenced by gender and age, with women being affected three times more often than men under the age of 40 years.[6] Another study by Blum et al performed a community-based survey of 165 Australians with a general practitioner confirming the diagnosis of MG. It was found that early onset of ages less than 40 years of age was more frequently female whereas late onset of MG over the age of 40 years was more frequently male.[10] It is important to question the reliability of the study due to the small sample population of the study. However, the results of this study had the same conclusion as the study by Gattellari.[7] Both the studies indicate that prevalence of MG was higher in women between ages 15 and 64 and higher in men over the age of 65.[7]

8.3.2 Determinants of Myasthenia Gravis

The precise cause of MG is unknown; however, abnormalities relating to the thymus gland (hyperplasia and neoplasia) have been shown to play a part in patients with anti-acetylcholine receptor antibodies as well as genetic predisposition which is likely to have an impact on the development of the disease.[6] Later onset after age 40 seems more likely to be a male patient and is usually reported to have normal thymic histology or thymic atrophy. More than 80% of those in early onset presented with positive anti-acetylcholine and thymic hyperplasia.[6] In addition, a systematic review by Carr et al described the influence of environmental and hormonal problems contributing to disease onset.[9]

A study performed by Blum et al found that factors that triggered and worsened MG included physical and emotional stress, infections, surgery, trauma, and medications.[10] They also found a cooccurrence of other immune-related diseases in 54% of the patients from the total of 165 Australian patients that they surveyed.[10] Moreover, the quality of life is severely affected by MG. Around 30% of the patients experience very severe symptoms that require hospitalization. Blum et al concluded that the factor associated with poor quality of life was depression where close to 40% experience it. Further, they have found that 40.6% of the 165 patients were working and 50% had required sick leave due to MG in the past 12 months.[10]

Patients incur financial pressure due to impact on employment and need for assistance daily. This has also been due to the impact of comorbidities in patients with MG. Study by Diaz and colleagues[11] concluded that out of the 253 patients, 73% were found to have comorbidities such as diabetes, hypertension, thymoma, and myasthenic crises. The study demonstrated that comorbidities are frequent in patients and may worsen the diagnosis of MG. It is recommended that patients with MG should be screened for diabetes, thyroid function, hypertension, and thymoma.[11]

8.4 Etiology and Pathogenesis of Myasthenia Gravis

The immune system is known for its role in defending the body against foreign organisms; however, occasionally it can counteract its normal function and turn against the host, resulting in an autoimmune disease.[12] In these disorders, immune cells that would typically attack microbes and pathogenic organisms erroneously attack the cells and/or proteins that have crucial roles in the body.[12] MG is a prototypical, autoimmune disease that is etiologically routed to the profile of the autoantibodies, the location of the affected muscles, the age of onset of symptoms, and thymic abnormalities.[4,13,14]

In the majority of reported MG cases, the immune system targets the nicotinic acetylcholine receptor (AChR), a membrane protein on muscle cells that is vital for muscle contraction (▶ Fig. 8.1).[4,15] It is indicated that at a normal NMJ, an active nerve cell prompts contraction

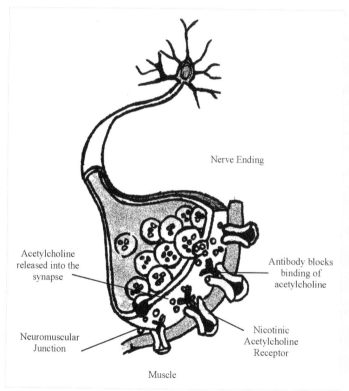

Fig. 8.1 Etiology of myasthenia gravis.

Nerve Ending

Acetylcholine released into the synapse

Antibody blocks binding of acetylcholine

Neuromuscular Junction

Nicotinic Acetylcholine Receptor

Muscle

of a muscle cell by releasing acetylcholine (ACh) from the motor nerve terminal in discrete packages (quanta).[13,15] The ACh quanta attaches to the AChR, a voltage-gated channel on the presynaptic terminal, generating an inward flux of ACh into the synaptic cleft that leads to the end-plate potential and gets hydrolyzed by acetylcholinesterase inside the synaptic cleft.[15,16] These contractions enable the individual to move a hand or complete any other voluntary movement.[15]

Commonly, 85% of the patients have antibodies against the nicotinic AChR present in their blood, and approximately 15% of individuals with MG are seronegative for antibodies to the AChR, implying that the antibodies are not identifiable in their serum.[14] However, recent studies have indicated that a small fraction of these individuals have antibodies to muscle-specific receptor kinase (MuSK) or the lipoprotein-related protein 4 (LRP4), a protein that assists in the arrangement of AChRs on the surface of the muscle cell.[6,13] In both instances, the binding of the pathogenic antibodies leads to a reduction of available protein receptors and impairs the neuromuscular transmission by complement-mediated damage of the receptors on the postsynaptic membrane.[17,18] While the underlying cause of MG remains unknown, several factors involving the induction and preservation of specific autoantigen responses that are observed in most striated muscles are broadly explored.

Moreover, the pathogenesis of MG depends upon the target and isotype of the antibodies. Most AChR antibodies belong to immunoglobulin (Ig) G1 and IgG3 (human) subclasses, which respond with various epitopes on the surfaces of AChRs.[4] Some antibodies stimulate, complement, and cause enzymatic lysis of the AChR on muscle cells; however, those that are exclusive to the key immunogenic region are more liable to crosslink the AChRs in the membrane and elevate their degradation rate, both mechanisms lead to the loss of AChR from the postsynaptic membrane.[4] The subsequent loss of AChRs at the NMJ impairs neuromuscular transmission, translating clinically to fatigue and muscle weakness.[4,16]

In the minority of patients, however, the autoantibodies bind to MuSK.[19] MuSK is a postsynaptic transmembrane tyrosine receptor kinase that is critical for the development and preservation of AChR at the NMJ.[20] MuSK forms the receptor configuration for agrin, a protein extant on synaptic basal lamina.[16] Interactions of Agrin/MuSK stimulate and preserve RAPSN-dependent clustering of AChR and other proteins present on the postsynaptic membrane.[21] RAPSN, present on the postsynaptic membrane, is a peripheral membrane protein essential for the clustering of AChR. Mice deficient in agrin or MuSK are unable to form NMJs and die at natal due to extreme muscle fatigue and weakness.[16,22] These antibodies are evidently pathogenic, but the mechanisms are only beginning to be understood.[15]

Furthermore, there is evidence that an immune regulator gland, thymus, is commonly associated with MG.[14] The thymus plays a critical part in the development of the immune system as it is responsible for producing a specific type of leukocytes, namely T-lymphocytes and T-cells, to defend the body from pathogenic organisms.[14,23] However, its role in the pathogenesis is highlighted by the assistance of thymectomy and the presence of recurrent histologic aberrations such as thymoma (benign or malignant) and follicular hyperplasia in the germinal center of the thymus.[23,24] This abnormality of the thymus gland leads to T-cells losing their capacity to distinguish between self and non-self, making them more probable to attack the body's normal cells.[25]

8.5 Genetic Component of Myasthenia Gravis

MG is a multifactorial disorder, significantly predisposed by genetic factors, even though it displays narrow scope for heritability.[26] MG predisposition has been investigated via family[27,28] and twin studies,[29] introspective of the disease's hereditary clustering and then of genetic inheritance. Bogdonas et al observed higher concordance values of MG among monozygotic twins than among dizygotic twins, strongly suggesting genetic interference in the pathogenesis of MG.[29] In addition, another study has reported that patients diagnosed with MG may be worsened with the presence of another autoimmune disease, most commonly, thyroid disorders and/or rheumatoid arthritis, indicating to the objective that a more generalized disturbance in the individual's immune system has occurred.[26]

Furthermore, in the onset of MG, the human leukocyte antigen (HLA) complex is implicated as a prominent involved genomic region. HLA-A1 and B8 alleles for the class I and DR3 for the class II encompass an inherited multigene haplotype termed "8.1" that has been reproducibly correlated with early onset MG and thymic hyperplasia.[30,31] In contrast to HLA, several HLA-unlinked genetic loci have also been explored with regards to their link to MG susceptibility.[26] In addition, other regulatory factors, genes, and cytokines, such as interferon regulatory factor 5, TNFα-induced protein 3, SNP rs13207033, and interleukin-10, all play a critical yet undefined role in immune system function.[19] The advancement of the human genome, genotyping, sequencing instruments, and the accessibility of statistical methods currently construct new possibilities in understanding the complex genome for variants influencing disease predisposition.[19]

8.6 Diagnostic Evaluation of Myasthenia Gravis

The defining characteristic of MG is fluctuating weakness and fatigue of skeletal muscles.[1] Signs and symptoms vary depending on the age of presentation and severity of the disease, including patterns of autoantibodies and associated thymic abnormalities (▸ Fig. 8.2). In more than 50% of cases, the initial presentation of MG involves ptosis and diplopia, resulting from weakness of the extraocular and levator palpebrae muscles.[32]

Weakness can remain localized in closely related muscle groups for long periods of time. For example, ocular myasthenia frequently affects the eye muscles, which occurs in roughly 15 to 20% of patients.[33] But it can also spread to other muscles, which is a condition termed *generalized MG*. The symptoms of generalized MG progress in a craniocaudal direction, the order being: from the ocular muscles, to the facial muscles to the lower bulbar muscles, to the truncal muscles, and finally to the limb muscles.[29] This occurs mostly within 2 years of the onset of the disease.[32]

Muscular weaknesses can lead to a plethora of related conditions. Dysphagia, dysarthria, and reduced facial expression (which often manifests as a snarling appearance when attempting to smile) can result from facial and masticatory muscular weakness.[33] Weakness in the soft palate and impaired lip movement may cause changes in phonation, usually with a nasal quality.[33] Weakness in the neck can cause problems such as head droop, and when the neck extensors are affected, the diaphragm is often affected. Severe cases may affect respiratory muscles to the point of myasthenic crisis, which is a respiratory collapse that can be fatal. It requires urgent treatment with mechanical ventilation.[33]

Much of muscular weaknesses are detectable on examination, but mild cases would necessitate tests of fatigue to be sure. Classic tests involve asking the patient to look up for several minutes (diagnosing ptosis or extraocular muscle weakness), repeatedly testing the strength of proximal muscles as well as counting aloud to 100 (listening for slurring or any exaggerated nasal quality in the voice).[33] These tests allow the physician to determine the severity and extent of the disease, in addition to providing feedback for implemented treatment plans. Diagnosis of MG in those patients presented with generalized muscle weakness that lacks ocular involvement, and with both normal sensory examination and deep tendon reflexes is always doubtful.[33]

Clinically a presentation of weakness and fatigability of skeletal muscles, with improvement after rest, is a rudimentary diagnostic test of MG.[33] The most touted diagnosis stems from detecting serum anti-acetylcholine receptor antibodies (AChK-ab).[34] These are found in 50 to 60% of patients with ocular MG and in 80 to 85% of patients with generalized MG.[34] An exception is an anti-AChR antibody,

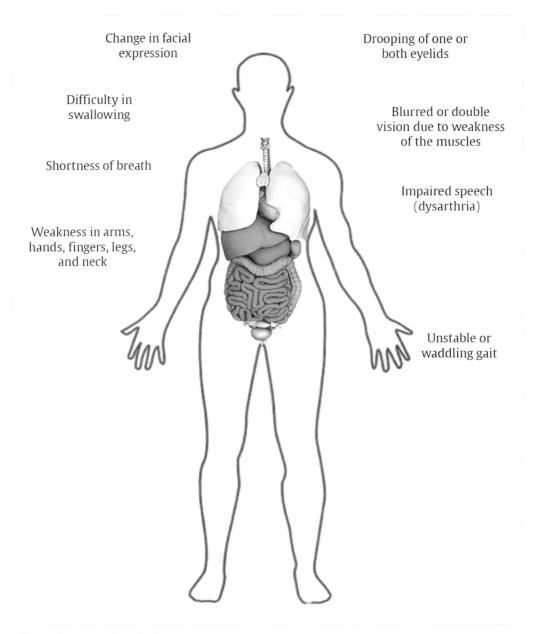

Change in facial expression

Drooping of one or both eyelids

Difficulty in swallowing

Blurred or double vision due to weakness of the muscles

Shortness of breath

Impaired speech (dysarthria)

Weakness in arms, hands, fingers, legs, and neck

Unstable or waddling gait

Fig. 8.2 Symptoms of myasthenia gravis.

the concentrations of which are unreliable indicators of the severity of MG. If anti-AChR antibodies are negative, the next step is to test anti-MuSK antibodies.[34] The seroconversion rate is 15% after 1 year for seronegative patients.[34] Immunosuppression can sometimes cause the disappearance of antibodies. Although some of these anti-striational anti-bodies can potentially indicate the disease prognosis and phenotype, the exact association has not yet fully elucidated.

In addition, diagnosis can also be aided by systemic administration of acetylcholinesterase inhibitors, known as the Tensilon test, which often uses neostigmine or edrophonium.[35] It aims to ascertain any reversibility of muscular weakness and can only be performed once that weakness has been confirmed. The sensitivity of the test peaks at 88% for generalized MG and 92% for ocular MG, with specificities of 97% for both disease forms.[35] However, it should be noted that false-positive edrophonium tests have been reported in various diseases, including non-neuromuscular diseases.[35] Hence, the diagnosis of MG has been a function of both clinical features and edrophonium responsiveness and other laboratory findings.

Electromyography studies have shown that repetitive nerve stimulation (RNS) is an effective technique for investigating neuromuscular transmission. However, its sensitivity can be relatively low, particularly for patients with mild symptoms and in those with anti-MuSK and MG.[36] Patients on chronically high doses of acetylcholinesterase inhibitors can also have misleading results.

Single-fiber electromyography (SFEMG), however, has shown impressive sensitivity, peaking at 99% for generalized MG and 80% for ocular MG and is always recommended in the diagnostic pathway for MG.[37] The specificity of SFEMG can be inconsistent; however, an atypical test can be demonstrated in other conditions such as mitochondrial cytopathy, motor neurone disease, or radiculopathy.[38]

8.7 Medical Management and Treatment of Myasthenia Gravis

A range of treatment modalities, alone or in combination, are used to alleviate symptoms of myasthenia gravis. These treatments include medications, intravenous therapy, and surgery (▶ Fig. 8.3). In addition, supplemental therapies such as a healthy diet, regular exercise, and stress management can assist in achieving more effective treatment results. The most appropriate treatment option is determined based on age, the severity of the condition, affected muscles, and other preexisting medical conditions.[39]

Two types of medications are used in the treatment of myasthenia gravis: cholinesterase inhibitors, which relieve symptoms temporarily, and immunosuppressants such as corticoids, which attack the source of the disease. The communication between nerves and muscles is enhanced by cholinesterase inhibitor medications such as pyridostigmine (Mestinon).[40] This is typically the first medication prescribed due to fewest long-term side effects and most rapid-acting mechanism. Breakdown of Ach, the chemical messenger of muscle contraction, is inhibited by these drugs. Although the underlying condition is not cured, the strength of contraction of the muscle can be improved. However, nausea, gastrointestinal upset, and excessive salivation and sweating may persist.[41] To attack the disease at its source, corticosteroids, such as prednisone, are used to inactivate the immune system, limiting antibody production. These drugs stop the body from degrading the NMJ by suppressing the body's immune system. Prolonged use of corticosteroids can increase the risk of infections and result in adverse effects such as bone thinning, diabetes, and weight gain.[42] Other immunosuppressants such as azathioprine (Imuran), cyclosporine (Sandimmune, Neoral), methotrexate (Trexall), mycophenolate mofetil (CellCept), or tacrolimus (Prograf) can also be used to alter the immune system. These immunosuppressants can also increase the risk of infections and have major adverse effects such as nausea, vomiting, gastrointestinal upset, liver damage, and kidney damage.[42]

Intravenous therapy consists of plasmapheresis, intravenous immunoglobulin (IVIg), and monoclonal antibody. Patients with severe MG symptoms who do not respond to other treatments or need to improve their strength before surgery can benefit from plasmapheresis.[43] In this treatment, a machine is used to filter out antibodies that block signal transmission from nerve endings to muscle receptor sites. The beneficial effects of this treatment, however, is generally temporary as it does not influence the ability to produce more antibodies. Heart rhythm problems, drop in blood pressure, bleeding, muscle cramps, or allergy to the plasma-replacing solutions are potential risks with this treatment.[44]

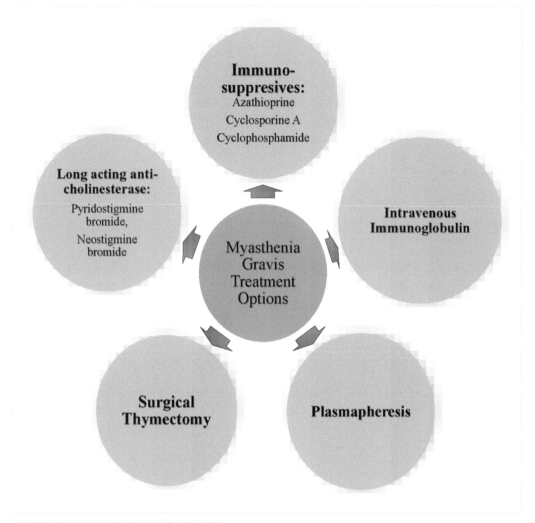

Fig. 8.3 Treatment options in myasthenia gravis.

Normal antibodies for the body are provided by the IVIg therapy, which alters the immune system response. It can only offer a short-duration relief from MG symptoms until longer acting immune-modifying treatments are affecting. IVIg is costly but has a lower potential of causing side effects in contrast to plasmapheresis and immune-suppressing therapy. The benefits, however, do not usually last more than a couple of weeks.[42] Headaches, chills, dizziness, and fluid retention are the possible side effects of this treatment. Monoclonal antibodies are antibodies that are made by identical immune cells and are clones of a unique parent cell. Monoclonal antibody Rituximab (Rituxan) is an intravenous medication, which acts by depleting certain white blood cells, hence altering the immune system. Rituximab is usually given at infusion centers or hospitals, and repeat infusions are often done over a few weeks.[45]

In the development of the immune system, the thymus gland plays a crucial role. This gland functions abnormally in about half of individuals suffering from MG. Thymectomy is the surgical removal of this gland. Tumors of the thymus gland are usually benign (thymoma), but in rare cases, they become malignant. Thymectomy is recommended for patients with thymoma; however, factors such as severity of the condition, sex, age, and the presence of AChR antibodies influence this treatment plan. This surgery could reduce the symptoms of MG symptoms or cure it through rebalancing the immune system. The results of this surgery are unpredictable and could take months to years to occur.[46] A thymectomy can be performed through minimally invasive or an open surgery. In a minimally invasive approach, the surgeon uses a smaller incision to utilize the video endoscopy and perform a robot-assisted thymectomy. The camera and mechanical arms of the robot system are used to increase precision and accuracy. As a result, this procedure reduces pain, blood loss, mortality rates, and hospital stays compared to open surgery.[47]

8.8 Management of a Dental Patient with Myasthenia Gravis

MG represents a challenge not only for the dentists but also the patients themselves. Indeed, the dental team should be cognizant of the precautions and modify the dental care to manage complications occurring in the dental office.[33] When handling a patient diagnosed with MG, there are several important factors that need to be considered.

The best dentistry is prevention! Every appointment that the patient walks into the dental office, they should be motivated in following good preventive oral care and dental hygiene at home. The weakness of the upper extremities and hand muscles and dysfunction of the facial muscles are common findings, resulting in a huge hurdle to maintaining a good oral hygiene at home, increasing the risk of infections of the oral cavity. It should be emphasized to start using an electric toothbrush or a manual toothbrush with a modified handle to minimize the muscle fatigue.[33] Chlorhexidine mouth rinse or gel may also be prescribed for preventing periodontal disease and are also acceptable for the myasthenic. However, it should be emphasized that the mouth rinses do not take the place of mechanical plaque control (brushing and flossing) and are merely an add-on.[3]

Myasthenic weakness can be worsened by oral infections and the psychological stress of undergoing dental treatment. That is why appointment scheduling plays a vital role in the management of the myasthenic patient. Dental appointments require using the facial muscles to keep the mouth open for lengthy periods, causing muscle fatigue, posing a challenge for MG patients. However, MG patients experience weakness of the muscles less in the morning than the rest of the day. Thus, the appointment should be short, and in the morning to reduce stress, minimize fatigue, and to take advantage of greater muscle strength. Also, mouth props can be used to minimize muscle strain while having to hold the mouth open during the treatment. However, remove the mouth prop periodically to provide the patient with a rest break and to avoid overstretching.[48]

Aspiration during dental treatment can be harmful to the human body, especially while applying restorative material such as amalgam, which has dangerous concentrations of mercury, a neurotoxin. Myasthenic patients may have developed a fear of choking since they have difficulty in swallowing. Impaired coughing reflex can worsen the threat of aspiration in these patients.[49] An additional factor that may increase the risk of increased aspiration of myasthenics during the appointment is due to the muscarinic side effect of anticholinesterase drug, as well as the use of mouth props. Hence, it is important to ensure efficient suction and the use of a rubber dam.[2]

The positioning of the patient on the dental chair is very crucial and should be carefully taken into consideration, especially if the patient has bulbar symptoms. The patient may feel safer and more comfortable in a semi-upright position (Fowler's position, where the head is raised 30–90 degrees above level), especially if he or she has trouble swallowing when in a supine position. Also, some patients may have MG condition affecting their palatal and pharyngeal muscles, causing regurgitation of fluids into the nose when swallowing. It would be wise to refer to a specialist in this situation. Patients with a disruptive gag reflex often find the treatment traumatizing and stressful—both psychologically and physiologically.[49] Thus, a supportive and open relationship should be established with the patient to lessen the emotional stress.[2]

Furthermore, it is worthwhile to realize that most MG patients have a well-controlled disease and with limited or no neuromuscular involvement, and thus, routine dental treatments and procedures such as root canals, fillings, etc. can safely be practiced in a private clinic. However, if a patient has frequent exacerbations or significant pharyngeal, respiratory, or generalized weakness, dental care should be provided in a hospital dental clinic or a facility with respiratory support capabilities and emergency intubation. A hospital dental clinic would also be preferred in situations requiring more advanced oral care such as oral surgery—multiple extractions, etc. Patient's medical history should also be examined, to check for frequent exacerbations, severe bulbar and respiratory symptoms, which would require the dentist to consult the patient's physician and a neurologist for an additional therapy before the treatment.[33]

8.8.1 Prior to and during Dental Treatment

Approximately 1 in 10,000 people carry the condition of MG, and therefore it is very likely that a dentist will encounter more than one patient present with this requiring some form of dental treatment.[50] This condition leads to weaknesses in facial muscles and the tongue, and this will inevitably impact the patient's oral hygiene and their capacity to wear dentures.[51] Furthermore, the medication taken by the patient for MG has the ability to interact with those given by the dentist.[3] These factors mean that the dentist should be aware of the way in which they will handle the patient both before and during the dental treatment.

Dental treatment with MG may be made difficult with the involvement of muscles, principally facial and masticatory ones.[2] Dentists have a duty to be aware of the medications in dentistry that can combat this aggravation of muscle weakness and fatigue that is characteristic of MG.[2] Dentists should also be able to adapt their treatment to deal with this muscular weakness and the medication therapy.

This involves determining and handling myasthenic dilemmas, averting the prospect of adverse drug interactions, and assessing the oral side effects of the medication and therapies that are utilized to treat MG. The use of the antibiotics that have muscle-relaxing ability (erythromycin, neomycin, and gentamicin), anesthesia, benzodiazepines, and sedation is contraindicated in patients with MG as these lead to further muscle weakness.[3] Only with the advice of a patient's physician should these be allowed. It is therefore imperative that there is contact between the dentist and other medical specialties concerning patients with this condition.

Contact between the dentist, patient, and even the neurologist is a necessity to prevent complications. Before their treatment, there has to be a complete examination of the symptoms for a patient with a known history of myasthenia. The patient's capacity to speak properly and swallow should also be assessed.[48]

For effective dental treatment, it is essential to realize that there exists a level of psychological stress that can lead to further myasthenic fatigue.[3] Shorter duration appointments in the morning will minimize this weakness, and the dentist can also use this to his convenience as muscle strength is greater in the morning.[48] Furthermore, the appointments should be scheduled at least 1 to 2 hours after the use of oral anticholinesterase medication. This helps in achieving the utmost therapeutic effect, thereby leading to a decline in the risk associated with myasthenic weakness.

The dentist should ensure that the patient arrives with time to spare for the appointment so that the patient can rest and refresh in an appropriately conditioned or ventilated office.[3] Preferably, a handicapped parking area close to the practice should be assigned to conserve the energy of the patient. The dentist is to bring the patient to a dental chair and allow the patient to have time there as opposed to sitting closely with other people in the waiting room.[16] Soothing music can be an option to further calm down the patient. The dentist should seek to build a relationship with the patient and reassure them of the treatment for the day. As is the norm for dental practice, all safety precautions including gloves and masks must be utilized.[2]

During the dental treatment, mouth props should be used to prevent the patient from muscle strain when they keep their mouth open for the treatment. If the patient has any problems with breathing, swallowing, or keeping their head up, the quantity of treatment, position of the chair, and the head support can all be utilized. If there are extreme cases with these issues, then the patients are best treated via dental hospitals or specialist offices. The myasthenic patient may have difficulty when reclining all the way back in the dental seat.[50] To refrain from the prospect of closing off the throat, a more upright position is recommended. A compromise between these positions is best to ensure that appropriate dental treatment can be undergone as well as that the patient feels comfortable in the position.

8.9 Oral Medicine Aspects of Myasthenia Gravis

Coordination between dentist, patient, and neurologist is necessary for delivering optimal dental treatment for a patient with myasthenia gravis. Appropriate considerations include drug interactions as well as procedural adjustments to accommodate the patient.[48] Numerous typical drugs used in dental treatment can aggravate the symptoms or cause further complications for MG patients, usually by exacerbating muscle weakness or interfering with respiration.

Corticosteroids are one class of drugs to treat MG, such as the immunosuppressant Prednisone. However, they may cause delayed healing and increase the risk of infection for wounds in the oral cavity. An antibiotic should thus be considered after relevant procedures such as those involving oral surgery. Cyclosporine, another immunosuppressant, can have interactions with common dental drugs that can cause increased kidney toxicity as well as elevated to possibly toxic levels of cyclosporine itself. Nephrotoxic interactions occur with antibiotics such as gentamicin, vancomycin, and antifungals such as ketoconazole as well as nonsteroidal anti-inflammatory drugs such as ibuprofen and Advil.[48] Cholinesterase inhibitors are another class of drugs used to treat MG. One such example is pyridostigmine, which may cause salivary gland stimulation to the point where it requires extra suctioning or even rubber dam isolation.

Procedural adjustments are necessary to avoid further complications during treatment. Oral anticholinesterases are recommended 1 to 2 hours before dental treatment to maximize their protective effects.[52] The use of bite blocks, rest periods, and other compensatory techniques should also be considered. Bilateral mandibular blocks should be avoided, however, as they may undermine the action of swallowing.[48] The dentist and patient must also find a compromise between comfort for swallowing and posture as well as access to deliver optimal dental care, as it is usually more difficult for the MG patient to lie back.[48] Sedation, typically with nitrous oxide, is a common approach to reduce the patient's stress and anxiety over dental treatment despite their condition.

Other drugs, relevant to consider, include aminoglycosides, which are a type of antibiotic that impairs neuromuscular transmission and creates dose-dependent muscular weakness (▶ Table 8.1). Also, anticonvulsants used in the treatment of epilepsy are contraindicated.[48] Local anesthetics are chosen over general anesthetics, and a vasoconstrictor is beneficial to increase the effects of the same dose.[49]

8.9.1 Coordination of Care between Dentist and Physician

MG requires close coordination of care between the patient's dentist and physician. This is due to a number of drug interactions

Table 8.1 A noncomprehensive table of drugs that are safe, that are to be used with caution, and that are contraindicated.[3]

Relatively contraindicated	Use with caution	Safe
Procaine	Lidocaine	
	Mepivacaine	
	Bupivacaine	
	Prilocaine	
	Morphine and derivatives	Acetaminophen
	Narcotics	NSAIDs
		Aspirin
	Benzodiazepines	N$_2$O/O$_2$ sedation
	Hypnotics	
	Barbiturates	
	Metronidazole	Penicillin and derivatives
Gentamycin		
Neomycin		
Polymixin B		
Bacitracin		
Clindamycin		
	Corticosteroids	

Abbreviation: NSAIDs, nonsteroidal anti-inflammatory drugs.

and special considerations before performing oral surgery. Being an autoimmune disease, patients may be treated with immunosuppressive drugs such as azathioprine, cyclophosphamide, and cyclosporine. Therefore, before performing oral surgery, there must be a collaboration with the physician as it may leave the patient with a high risk of infection, as well as delayed wound healing due to immune suppression. Following surgery, a course of antibiotics should be considered to help minimize the risk of infection. Prednisone is another immunosuppressive drug that requires special consideration prior to stressful or complicated dental procedures. Prednisone is a corticosteroid that, at high doses, may lead to adrenal gland suppression affecting the adrenal glands' ability to respond to stress.[53] Thus, coordination between patient and dentist is important to decide whether additional steroid supplements are required before more invasive and stressful procedures.

A level of collaboration between physician and oral health practitioner is also required when considering which antibiotic is most appropriate. Tetracycline, aminoglycosides, and erythromycin are examples of antibiotics that have muscle relaxant properties. They work by inhibiting the release of ACh from the presynaptic terminal, stabilizing the postsynaptic membrane.[48] In the case of patients with MG, these antibiotics should be avoided. In addition, fluoroquinolones must also be avoided, as there is a chance of prolonged myasthenic crisis after administration.[54]

Aside from these considerations of antibiotics and immunosuppressive drugs, careful control of anesthetics must be exercised when dealing with such patients. Local anesthetics are much more suitable over general anesthesia for a myasthenic patient. Lidocaine has the potential of exacerbating MG intravenously; however, if required locally, it may be used with caution. Mepivicaine, on the other hand, may be a better choice as it has few side effects and has a shorter duration.[55] Local infiltration, intraligamentary, and intrapulpal injection techniques can be used to help reduce the dose of local anesthetic in preference to nerve block anesthesia.[48] Oral practitioners, with patients that experience recurrent, severe exacerbations of weakness from the autoimmune disease, should consult the physician to consider additional myasthenic therapy (such as plasma exchange) prior to oral surgery.[56] Furthermore, coordination is required where the patient's exchange protocol requires anticoagulants, such as heparin. In such cases, oral practitioners should ensure dental treatment dates do not coincide with exchange days in the patient's treatment sequence.

MG patients present many challenges to the dental profession as a result of the head, neck, and oral regions being affected. Developing a treatment plan requires sufficient knowledge about the condition and the limitations it inflicts on not only the patient but the oral health care provider. Thorough attention to medications, signs and symptoms, method, and timing of treatment and comprehensive knowledge about the nature of the disease are vital to avoid any complications. In coordination with physicians, dentists who are aware of the management of this disease can safely and effectively provide MG patients appropriate oral health care.

References

[1] McCullough M. Treatment of myasthenia gravis. Aust Prescr. 2007; 30(6)

[2] Yarom N, Barnea E, Nissan J, Gorsky M. Dental management of patients with myasthenia gravis: a literature review. Oral Surg Oral Med Oral Pathol Oral Radiol Endod. 2005; 100(2): 158–163

[3] Patton LL, Howard JF, Jr. Myasthenia gravis: dental treatment considerations. Spec Care Dentist. 1997; 17(1):25–32

[4] Phillips WD, Vincent A. Pathogenesis of myasthenia gravis: update on disease types, models, and mechanisms. F1000 Res. 2016; 5:F1000

[5] Rapoport H, Popko M, Findler M, Findler M. Dental treatment for patients with myasthenia gravis. Refuat Hapeh Vehashinayim. 2005; 22(3):35–40

[6] Meriggioli MN, Sanders DB. Autoimmune myasthenia gravis: emerging clinical and biological heterogeneity. Lancet Neurol. 2009; 8(5):475–490

[7] Gattellari M, Goumas C, Worthington JM. A national epidemiological study of myasthenia gravis in Australia. Eur J Neurol. 2012; 19(11):1413–1420

[8] McGrogan A, Sneddon S, de Vries CS. The incidence of myasthenia gravis: a systematic literature review. Neuroepidemiology. 2010; 34(3):171–183

[9] Carr AS, Cardwell CR, McCarron PO, McConville J. A systematic review of population based epidemiological studies in myasthenia gravis. BMC Neurol. 2010; 10:46

[10] Blum S, Lee D, Gillis D, McEniery DF, Reddel S, McCombe P. Clinical features and impact of myasthenia gravis disease in Australian patients. J Clin Neurosci. 2015; 22(7): 1164–1169

[11] Cacho Diaz B, Flores-Gavilán P, García-Ramos G. Myasthenia gravis and its comorbidities. J Neurol Neurophysiol. 2015; 06 (05)

[12] Nicholson LB. The immune system. Essays Biochem. 2016; 60 (3):275–301

[13] Turner C. A review of myasthenia gravis: pathogenesis, clinical features and treatment. Curr Anaesth Crit Care. 2007; 18 (1):15–23

[14] Berrih-Aknin S, Frenkian-Cuvelier M, Eymard B. Diagnostic and clinical classification of autoimmune myasthenia gravis. J Autoimmun. 2014; 48–49:143–148

[15] Giraud M, Vandiedonck C, Garchon HJ. Genetic factors in autoimmune myasthenia gravis. Ann N Y Acad Sci. 2008; 1132(1):180–192

[16] Jayam Trouth A, Dabi A, Solieman N, Kurukumbi M, Kalyanam J. Myasthenia gravis: a review. Autoimmune Dis. 2012; 2012: 874680

[17] Avidan N, Le Panse R, Berrih-Aknin S, Miller A. Genetic basis of myasthenia gravis - a comprehensive review. J Autoimmun. 2014; 52:146–153

[18] Vincent A. Unravelling the pathogenesis of myasthenia gravis. Nat Rev Immunol. 2002; 2(10):797–804

[19] Zagoriti Z, Georgitsi M, Giannakopoulou O, et al. Genetics of myasthenia gravis: a case-control association study in the Hellenic population. Clin Dev Immunol. 2012; 2012:484919

[20] Hubbard SR, Gnanasambandan K. Structure and activation of MuSK, a receptor tyrosine kinase central to neuromuscular junction formation. Biochim Biophys Acta. 2013; 1834(10): 2166–2169

[21] Hughes BW, Kusner LL, Kaminski HJ. Molecular architecture of the neuromuscular junction. Muscle Nerve. 2006; 33(4): 445–461

[22] Conti-Fine BM, Milani M, Kaminski HJ. Myasthenia gravis: past, present, and future. J Clin Invest. 2006; 116(11):2843–2854

[23] Le Panse R, Bismuth J, Cizeron-Clairac G, et al. Thymic remodeling associated with hyperplasia in myasthenia gravis. Autoimmunity. 2010; 43(5–6):401–412

[24] Marx A, Pfister F, Schalke B, Saruhan-Direskeneli G, Melms A, Ströbel P. The different roles of the thymus in the pathogenesis of the various myasthenia gravis subtypes. Autoimmun Rev. 2013; 12(9):875–884

[25] Romi F. Thymoma in myasthenia gravis: from diagnosis to treatment. Autoimmune Dis. 2011; 2011:474512

[26] Christensen PB, Jensen TS, Tsiropoulos I, et al. Associated autoimmune diseases in myasthenia gravis: a population-based study. Acta Neurol Scand. 1995; 91(3):192–195

[27] Marrie RA, Sahlas DJ, Bray GM. Familial autoimmune myasthenia gravis: four patients involving three generations. Can J Neurol Sci. 2000; 27(4):307–310

[28] Namba T, Brunner NG, Brown SB, Muguruma M, Grob D. Familial myasthenia gravis. Report of 27 patients in 12 families and review of 164 patients in 73 families. Arch Neurol. 1971; 25(1):49–60

[29] Bogdanos DP, Smyk DS, Rigopoulou EI, et al. Twin studies in autoimmune disease: genetics, gender and environment. J Autoimmun. 2012; 38(2–3):J156–J169

[30] Horton R, Gibson R, Coggill P, et al. Variation analysis and gene annotation of eight MHC haplotypes: the MHC Haplotype Project. Immunogenetics. 2008; 60(1):1–18

[31] Giraud M, Beaurain G, Yamamoto AM, et al. Linkage of HLA to myasthenia gravis and genetic heterogeneity depending on anti-titin antibodies. Neurology. 2001; 57(9):1555–1560

[32] Nair AG, Patil-Chhablani P, Venkatramani DV, Gandhi RA. Ocular myasthenia gravis: a review. Indian J Ophthalmol. 2014; 62(10):985–991

[33] Tamburrini A, Tacconi F, Barlattani A, Mineo TC. An update on myasthenia gravis, challenging disease for the dental profession. J Oral Sci. 2015; 57(3):161–168

[34] Hilton-Jones D. Diagnose myasthenia gravis. Pract Neurol. 2002; 3:173–177

[35] Mehndiratta MM, Pandey S, Kuntzer T. Acetylcholinesterase Inhibitor Treatment for Myasthenia Gravis. Cochrane Database of Systematic Reviews. John Wiley & Sons, Ltd; 2011

[36] Kim SW, Sunwoo MK, Kim SM, Shin HY, Sunwoo IN. Repetitive nerve stimulation in MuSK-antibody-positive myasthenia gravis. J Clin Neurol. 2017; 13(3):287–292

[37] Oh SJ, Kim DE, Kuruoglu R, Bradley RJ, Dwyer D. Diagnostic sensitivity of the laboratory tests in myasthenia gravis. Muscle Nerve. 1992; 15(6):720–724

[38] Sathasivam S. Diagnosis and management of myasthenia gravis. Prog Neurol Psychiatry. 2014; 18(1):6–14

[39] Pevzner A, Schoser B, Peters K, et al. Anti-LRP4 autoantibodies in AChR- and MuSK-antibody-negative myasthenia gravis. J Neurol. 2012; 259(3):427–435

[40] Fambrough DM, Drachman DB, Satyamurti S. Neuromuscular junction in myasthenia gravis: decreased acetylcholine receptors. Science. 1973; 182(4109):293–295

[41] Colović MB, Krstić DZ, Lazarević-Pašti TD, Bondžić AM, Vasić VM. Acetylcholinesterase inhibitors: pharmacology and toxicology. Curr Neuropharmacol. 2013; 11(3):315–335

[42] Kraker J, Zivković SA. Autoimmune neuromuscular disorders. Curr Neuropharmacol. 2011; 9(3):400–408

[43] Jolles S, Sewell WA, Misbah SA. Clinical uses of intravenous immunoglobulin. Clin Exp Immunol. 2005; 142(1):1–11

[44] Hartung HP, Mouthon L, Ahmed R, Jordan S, Laupland KB, Jolles S. Clinical applications of intravenous immunoglobulins (IVIg): beyond immunodeficiencies and neurology. Clin Exp Immunol. 2009; 158 Suppl 1:23–33

[45] Nowak RJ, Dicapua DB, Zebardast N, Goldstein JM. Response of patients with refractory myasthenia gravis to rituximab: a retrospective study. Ther Adv Neurol Disorder. 2011; 4(5):259–266

[46] Taioli E, Paschal PK, Liu B, Kaufman AJ, Flores RM. Comparison of Conservative treatment and thymectomy on myasthenia gravis outcome. Ann Thorac Surg. 2016; 102(6):1805–1813

[47] Veronesi G, Novellis P, Voulaz E, Alloisio M. Robot-assisted surgery for lung cancer: state of the art and perspectives. Lung Cancer. 2016; 101:28–34

[48] Patil PM, Singh G, Patil SP. Dentistry and the myasthenia gravis patient: a review of the current state of the art. Oral Surg Oral Med Oral Pathol Oral Radiol. 2012; 114(1):e1–e8

[49] Lotia S, Randall C, Dawson LJ, Longman LP. Dental management of the myasthenic patient. Dent Update. 2004; 31(4):237–242

[50] Lynn S. Treating patients with myasthenia gravis. Dimens Dent Hyg. 2013; 11(8):14–18

[51] Gilhus NE. Myasthenia gravis. N Engl J Med. 2016; 375(26):2570–2581

[52] Rai B. Myasthenia gravis: challenge to dental profession. Internet J Acad Physician Assist 2006;6(1): 1–4

[53] Gibson N, Ferguson JW. Steroid cover for dental patients on long-term steroid medication: proposed clinical guidelines based upon a critical review of the literature. Br Dent J. 2004; 197(11):681–685

[54] Jones SC, Sorbello A, Boucher RM. Fluoroquinolone-associated myasthenia gravis exacerbation: evaluation of postmarketing reports from the US FDA adverse event reporting system and a literature review. Drug Saf. 2011; 34(10):839–847

[55] Abel M, Eisenkraft JB. Anesthetic implications of myasthenia gravis. Mt Sinai J Med. 2002; 69(1–2):31–37

[56] Kumar R, Birinder SP, Gupta S, Singh G, Kaur A. Therapeutic plasma exchange in the treatment of myasthenia gravis. Indian J Crit Care Med. 2015; 19(1):9–13

9 Facial Paralysis

Armin Ariana

Abstract

The facial nerve carries the motor fibers for the facial expression and mastication and the sensory fibers to the external ear and the special sensation of taste. Partial weakening or loss of function of the facial nerve due to paralysis, therefore, affects innervated structures and associated functions depending on where the paralysis of the facial nerve is located. This can be presented as a unilateral or bilateral loss of voluntary and involuntary facial muscle movements. An asymmetric smile, dry eyes, involuntary muscle movements, reduced tolerance to sounds, abnormal blinking, issues in speech articulation, involuntary drooling, alterations in taste perception, and facial pain are some of the symptoms of such paralysis. With a broad management variability, health practitioners initially investigate the etiological nature of the condition. An oral health practitioner can encounter a patient with a facial paralysis, be the first one to diagnose a patient with facial paralysis or induce facial paralysis iatrogenically during simple or complex dental procedures. It is therefore important to involve the medical practitioner and relevant medical specialties in determining and confirming the specific cause and etiology of the facial paralysis as it may be multifactorial and require treatment from other disciplines in order to provide the best possible outcome for the patient.

Keywords: facial palsy, epidemiology, pathogenesis, treatment, oral manifestations, medical management

9.1 Background of Facial Paralysis

The facial nerve (cranial nerve VII) is composed of two roots, a motor and sensory root.[1] The large motor root carries the motor fibers to the muscles of facial expression and mastication. The sensory root carries general sensory fibers to parts of the external ear and the special sensation of taste to the anterior two-thirds of the tongue and the palate. The sensory root contains some parasympathetic secretomotor fibers as well which supply the submandibular and sublingual salivary glands, as well as the lacrimal glands and the minor mucous glands of the nose and palate. Since facial paralysis causes the partial weakening or loss of function of the facial nerve due to the cessation or inhibition of nerve impulse propagation,[1] any structures and their associated functions innervated by the facial nerve can also be affected depending on where the paralysis of the facial nerve is located.

Facial paralysis presents as a unilateral or bilateral loss of voluntary and nonvoluntary facial muscle movements. This can cause symptoms such as an asymmetric smile, dry eyes, involuntary muscle movements, reduced tolerance to sounds, abnormal blinking, issues in speech articulation, involuntary drooling, alterations in taste perception, and facial pain.[2] Since symptoms cause deficiencies in taste, mastication, speaking, and expressing emotions, the patient's physical and emotional health is affected.[3]

Management for facial paralysis can vary broadly. This is due to the complex etiological nature of the condition. There are a number of known causes for facial paralysis, the most common being Bell palsy, an idiopathic disease that can only be diagnosed by exclusion. Treatment plans differ, depending on cause and severity of injury.[4] Bell palsy presents as unilateral drooping of the face. An asymmetrically sloping mouth is the landmark feature of Bell palsy. Bell palsy is a peripheral paralysis of the 7th cranial nerve. Central paralyses can occur as well, often as a result of a stroke. Central and peripheral palsies present differently. Central paralysis only involves the unilateral side of the lower face while peripheral palsy most commonly affects the entire, unilateral side of the face.[5]

9.2 Description of Facial Paralysis

Paralysis of the face has been an observed phenomenon for millennia. Ancient Greek, Roman, Egyptian, and Persian cultures all have documented conditions that resemble facial paralysis.[6] Hippocrates was one of the earliest to record such conditions. In his writings from around the fifth century BCE, he vaguely described distortions of the face that would resolve without treatment.[7]

For a long time Charles Bell was credited with the first comprehensive description of idiopathic facial paralysis in 1821, hence its name Bell palsy.[6] However, it was later discovered that a number of individuals before Bell recorded accounts of facial paralysis.[8] The first comprehensive account of facial paralysis is that of the Persian Physician known as Razi. In his sixth book of al-Hawi, Razi was able to differentiate between facial nerve spasms, central paralysis, and peripheral paralysis. Razi is credited with being the first to describe the clinical features of Bell palsy. His findings were documented around the ninth century CE.[9] Dutchman Cornelis Stalpart van der Wiel is now largely regarded as the first to comprehensively document the clinical features of Bell palsy, rather than Charles Bell himself. He described the palsy as being one-sided and healing in several weeks without treatment. He documented this description in 1683 in his second publication of "Hundred Rare Observations."[10] Following Stalpart van der Wiel, Nikolaus Anton Friedreich (1798) and James Douglas (1704) also appear to have observed and described facial paralysis before Bell in the 18th century.[11]

9.3 Epidemiology of Facial Paralysis

Facial paralysis varies depending on the level of facial nerve lesion. This phenomenon can be reversed spontaneously or via clinical or surgical treatment. About 20% of patients develop some form of sequelae, with unilateral and bilateral complete paralysis of facial muscle movements being the most severe outcome.[3] The global annual incidence of facial paralysis is approximately 70 cases per 100,000 population. In a study published by Bleicher et al, the global annual number of cases of permanent facial paralysis was estimated to be 127,000.[12] The prevalence, which refers to the number of existing cases or lesions within a defined population at a specific point in time,[13] of facial paralysis, was greater among patients that are younger than 20.[3] Also, according to a study conducted at Murtala Muhammed Specialist Hospital, Kano, Nigeria between January 2000 and December 2005,[14] males had a higher incidence of facial paralysis than females at 56.2%, it was most common among businessmen at 31.6%, and that right-sided facial palsy was slightly more predominant compared to the left.

Facial paralysis remains a challenge diagnostically due to the high number of causes. Multiple causes of facial paralysis have been described in the literature. In two-thirds of the cases studied, the cause is unknown and are referred to as idiopathic paralysis or Bell palsy.[3] In the United States, the annual incidence, which refers to the number of new cases or lesions of a specific disease arising over a given period of time within a specified population,[13] of Bell palsy is approximately 23 cases per 100,000 population. Bell palsy is thought to account for approximately 60 to 75% cases of acute unilateral facial paralysis.[15] Hence, Bell palsy is the most common cause of facial nerve paralysis. However, there are many other causes for facial paralysis that makes up for the remaining one-third of the cases. All the major causes will be explained in detail later in subsequent sections, but for now, the distribution of facial paralysis by cause shall be discussed. According to a retrospective study by Batista (2011), 122 (42.8%) of the patients admitted to the hospital with facial paralysis were due to Bell palsy characteristics, 54 (18.9%) due to stroke, 48 (16.8%) due to congenital paralysis, 9 (3.2%) due to facial trauma, 17 (6%) due to traumatic brain injuries, 7 (2.4%) due to vestibular schwannoma, 9 (3.2%) due to tumors, and 19 (6.7%) due to other etiologies (▶ Fig. 9.1).[3]

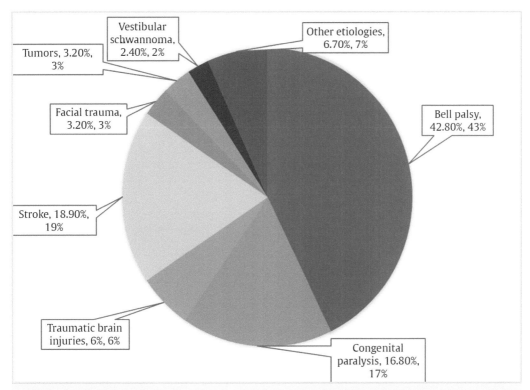

Fig. 9.1 Processed quantitative data showing the percentage of patients diagnosed with facial paralysis due to Bell palsy, congenital paralysis, traumatic brain injuries, stroke, facial trauma, tumors, vestibular schwannoma, and other etiologies admitted to the study of Batista in 2011.[3]

In an attempt to explain the differences in these values between the different causes of facial paralysis (analytical epidemiology), Bell palsy (most common) and other causes of facial paralysis, which are less common, are compared. Bell palsy is significantly higher than other causes (42.80% compared to second most common 16.80% in congenital paralysis) because there are many factors that lead to Bell palsy in comparison to other causes: Bell palsy occurs when the nerves of facial muscles become compressed or inflamed, when viral infection such as viral meningitis or herpes simplex are present, and also when associated with diabetes, chronic middle ear infection, headaches, influenza, tumors, high blood pressure, Lyme disease, sarcoidosis, and facial trauma.[16] The second most common congenital paralysis in comparison is only affected by traumatic injury or developmental deformities of the brain or cranial nerve VII of the facial nerve.[17]

9.4 Etiology and Pathogenesis of Facial Paralysis

The most commonly diagnosed cause of facial paralysis is Bell palsy (▶ Fig. 9.2).[18] This condition is poorly understood and often thought to be of idiopathic origin and thus diagnosed by exclusion.[19] However, recent scientific advances have and are still exploring a possible link between numerous infectious agents and Bell palsy, but as this is not completely understood yet, they will be handled separately, given the assumption that a causal relationship does not exist between them.[20]

Some of these infectious agents leading to the development of facial paralysis include varicella zoster virus; herpes simplex virus; spirochete *Borrelia burgdorferi* giving rise to Lyme disease; and *Streptococcus pneumonia*, *Haemophilus influenzae*, and *Moraxella catarrhalis* as the most frequent causative agents of otitis media.[19]

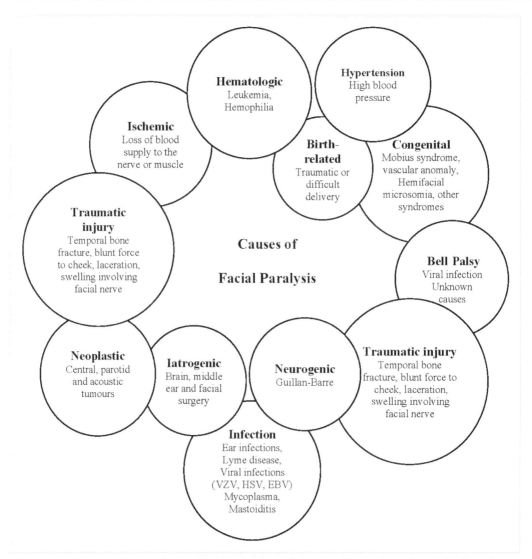

Fig. 9.2 Causes of facial palsy.

The varicella zoster virus is a member of the Herpesviridae family and following the primary varicella infection establishes a ganglionic latency.[21] When this latency is established in the sensory fibers of the geniculate ganglion, reactivation of the virus, often precipitated by factors including stress, trauma, and immune deficiency, results in Ramsay Hunt syndrome type 2.[16] This reactivation as herpes zoster leads to inflammation in the geniculate ganglion, and it is this inflammation that results in disrupted motor function of the facial nerve as visceral efferent

fibers from the motor nucleus of CN VII pass through the geniculate ganglion and are thus affected.[22] In addition, visceral afferent taste fibers from the anterior two-thirds of the tongue and visceral efferent parasympathetic fibers that innervate the salivary and lacrimal glands are affected as they also pass through the geniculate ganglion leading to decreased taste sensation, salivation, and lacrimation.[22]

The herpes simplex virus (HSV) is another member of the Herpesviridae family and, similar to the varicella zoster virus, establishes latency following primary infection.[23] HSV-1 is most often associated with cold sores and HSV-2 with genital herpes. The virus lies dormant in peripheral nerve cell axons and when activated leads to an inflammation of the endoneurium and demyelination of the nerve fiber.[19] Facial nerve demyelination leads to slower conduction of action potentials along the axon of the nerve fiber and depending on the extent of the demyelination, paralysis. Moreover, when the endoneuritis spreads to the facial canal, facial nerve paralysis results from the compression of the nerve due to the local swelling.[24]

Lyme disease is spread through vector-borne transmission, primarily ticks, and is classified into acute and chronic stages of the disease, both of which represent periods for facial nerve paralysis to occur.[25] When the spirochete bacteria directly invade the nervous system, neural abnormalities develop.[19] One such abnormality, cranial neuralgia, which has been found to manifest within 2 days to 2 months of illness, may result in the paralysis of any cranial nerve.[25] When this neuralgia affects the facial nerve, facial paralysis results.

Otitis media is an infection of the middle ear. While facial nerve paralysis is an important complication, little is understood on the mechanism through which this palsy results.[26] In acute otitis media, facial paralysis is believed to be a consequence of bacterial toxins associated with the infection affecting the facial nerve in the facial canal and resulting in inflammatory edema.[27] In chronic suppurative otitis media, it is thought that facial paralysis may be a result of either the spreading of the body's chronic inflammatory response from the middle ear to the facial nerve or from direct pressure on the facial nerve by a pathology, most frequently a cholesteatoma.[28]

Another cause of facial paralysis is stroke. Ischemic stroke occurs because of an inadequate supply of blood and oxygen to tissue in the brain and it is in this ischemic environment that the brain cells cease to function and may die if deprived of oxygen for too long. Hence it is the location of the ischemia that will determine whether the facial nerve is affected and the duration that will determine whether facial paralysis results.[29] In hemorrhagic stroke, it is the rupture of a blood vessel in the brain and the subsequent bleeding that may cause facial paralysis depending on whether the bleeding is placing pressure on the facial nerve.[30]

Facial paralysis may also be a result of a tumor either growing within the nerve or compressing the nerve anywhere along its course.[20] Neoplasms of the parotid gland, most often adenoid cystic carcinoma, are one such source through which facial paralysis may manifest.[31] Paralysis is a result of the expansion of the neoplasm within the parotid gland leading to either compression of the nerve with subsequent ischemia or perineural invasion.[31,32] The part of the nerve that is paralyzed will depend on the location of the neoplasm within the gland.

Trauma is another origin from which facial paralysis can develop.[20] Of particular dental relevance is the trauma to the facial nerve sustained during dental surgery.[33] When performing an inferior alveolar nerve block as part of a dental surgery, it is the close association between the inferior alveolar nerve and the facial nerve that makes physical trauma to the facial nerve by the needle a possibility.[34] Traumatizing the facial nerve, through perforating it with the needle, results in facial paralysis.[35] It has also been suggested that the deposition of lignocaine into or around the nerve, by injecting into the parotid gland, may lead to local anesthetic toxicity of the facial nerve and thus paralysis.[34]

Genetic syndromes may also play a role in the development of facial paralysis. These include Melkersson-Rosenthal syndrome, Albers-Schönberg disease (osteopetrosis), Möbius syndrome, and Goldenhar syndrome (oculoauriculovertebral dysplasia).[19] The summary of causes of facial paralysis is presented in ▶ Fig. 9.3.

9.5 Genetic Component of Facial Paralysis

9.5.1 Möbius Syndrome

Möbius syndrome (MBS) is a rare congenital condition that affects every 1 in 50,000 live

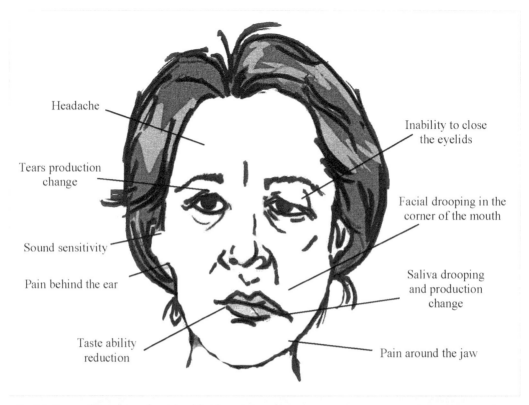

Fig. 9.3 Signs and symptoms of peripheral facial paralysis.

births. The clinical findings of MBS can vary significantly in terms of both symptoms and their severity. However, one typical characteristic involves the paralysis of the facial (VII) nerve either unilaterally or bilaterally. The most widely accepted theory regarding facial paralysis from MBS is thought to occur due to an interruption to vascular supply leading to ischemia and malformation of the facial nerve. Recent studies have produced findings which indicate that MBS may result from rhomben-cephalon developmental defects rather than isolated facial nerve dysfunction as in hereditary congenital facial palsy (HCFP).[36]

FLTI/VEGFR1 is one gene thought to be involved in abnormal vascular growth, associated with MBS and resulting facial paralysis.[36] Mutations in two homeobox genes, *HOXA1* and *HOXB1*, also have been found to contain overlapping features with MBS. These said mutations produce phenotypes that are typical of MBS including facial weakness, indicat-

ing an association with the syndrome.[37] Two genes, *PLXND1* and *REV3L*, present within the HCFP1 and HCFP2 loci, respectively, have been confirmed to be associated with MBS. *PLXND1* encodes for a multitude of amino acids, and mutations to this gene cause defects in moto-neuron migration, affecting neural fiber structures. The gene *REV3L* is associated with hypoplasia of neural structures in mice and is also linked to DNA damage.[38]

9.5.2 Goldenhar Syndrome (Oculoauriculovertebral Dysplasia)

Goldenhar syndrome is congenital defect with incidence of 1 in 5000 to 25,000 live births with a prevalence in males. Facial nerve palsy is one characteristic associated with the typical craniofacial abnormalities found in Goldenhar syndrome, although this has not been confirmed and remains largely unstudied.[39]

9.5.3 Albers-Schonberg Disease (Osteopetrosis)

Albers-Schonberg disease is a disorder of autosomal dominance and is the most common type of osteopetrosis, a disease that affects the functioning ability of the body's osteoclasts.[40] This disease typically onsets during adulthood with a defect in the osteoclast's ability for resorption, resulting in increased mass of skeletal bone. Facial nerve paralysis of bilateral range typically arises in Albers-Schonberg disease due to facial canal stenosis, leading to ischemia or rupture of the facial canal due to overgrowth of the epitympanum.[41] Recent studies have confirmed that mutations in the genes encoding for ClCN7 chloride channels on chromosome 16p13.3 are responsible for Albers-Schonberg disease. This chloride channel allows for osteoclasts to resorb bone through acidification of the extracellular lacuna and ceases to function in patients with this disease.[40]

9.5.4 Melkersson-Rosenthal Syndrome

Melkersson-Rosenthal syndrome (MRS) is a rare, granulomatous disorder that may present with intermittent or relapsing facial paralysis. This disease typically onsets at 25 years old; however, it can affect all age groups.[42] Although much of the genetics remains relatively unknown, studies have been conducted showing a hereditary link between those with existing MRS and a familial history of facial palsy. Further study in 2015 implicated that MRS-induced facial palsy is of autosomal-recessive inheritance.[43]

9.5.5 Hereditary Congenital Facial Paresis

Hereditary congenital facial paresis (HCFP) is an autosomal-dominant disorder that exists separately from the previously mentioned genetic syndromes.[44] This disease is classified as a congenital cranial dysinnervation disorder (CCDD) alongside MBS and is characterized by weakness or paralysis of the facial muscles and dysfunction of the facial nerve (CN VII). However, unlike MBS, the paralysis results from either unilateral or bilateral malformation of the facial branchiomotor (FBM) nucleus.[17]

There are three genetic subdivisions of this disease: HFCP1, HFCP2, and HFCP3, the latter of which has only recently been discovered. The former two subtypes were initially thought to be subtypes of MBS. However, this has been proved to be incorrect, and the loci suggested to be associated with the syndrome on chromosomes 3q21.2-q22.1 and 10q21.3-q22.1 have now been renamed from MBS2 and MBS3 to HFCP1 and HFCP2. Studies have been conducted to identify genes from the mentioned loci that are involved in HCFP. From the HFCP1 and HFCP2 loci, three genes have been shown to display expressional associations to FBM nucleus development. MgII is one the first loci that codes for lipase and is expressed in zones that largely coincide with the migratory route of facial motoneurons, indicating an association. The two suggested associated genes from HCFP2 are REEP3 and LRRTM3. REEP3 has shown expression in the FBM nucleus, and mutations to certain segments of REEP3 are known to be associated with other diseases such as autism. In contrast, LRRTM3 is involved with development of neurons, hence possibly relatable to the facial nerve. However, it is necessary to conduct further studies in order to prove its role in the specific development of the FBM.[17] From the HCFP3 locus, the gene *HOXB1*, which also correlates to MBS, has been indicated to be associated with HCFP, where mutations in the Arg5 homeodomain are thought to be responsible.[44]

9.6 Diagnostic Evaluation of Facial Paralysis

Identification of facial paralysis is mostly done clinically. There are factors that act as a good indicator of facial paralysis such as facial drooping, eyelid weakness, puffing out the cheeks, and raising both eyebrows. In facial paralysis, there are two types of lesions, which are central and peripheral. The central lesion, which is a stroke, spares forehead and drooping lips whereas peripheral lesion, which is Bell palsy, leads to patients not being able to spare forehead but droops forehead and lips.[45]

The physical examination should include a complete head-and-neck examination with an emphasis on ear, mastoid, and parotid glands. When performing the physical examination, it is necessary to assess the patient's motor function.[46] Thus consider if the patient has peripheral facial palsy, if the patient closes the eyes tightly, if the smile is symmetric, if the patient is able to puff out the cheeks, and such, because most of the times with facial paralysis patients, they present difficulties doing those movements.[45]

Medical history of patients provides clues to narrow the differential diagnosis.[46] When examining an acute event, there are a couple of factors to be considered; duration of paralysis, onset time, past history of facial paralysis, the presence of skin rashes, and any potential tick exposure. For example, if the patient has gone camping and could have been tick-exposed, the patient could be suspicious of Lyme disease causing the facial paralysis.[47]

In relation to the facial paralysis caused by Lyme disease, people who live in an area where Lyme disease is endemic are likely to be exposed to ticks, which can lead to facial paralysis. In this case, patients will need to have a laboratory testing to further investigate. How the testing works is that patients would have to have the enzyme-linked immunosorbent assay run for the screening of the disease of interest. However, other options are possible, which is the indirect fluorescent antibody test to do so. In case of a positive result from the assay, the diagnosis of Lyme disease will have to be double-checked by protein immunoblot known as Western blot.[47]

For other differential diagnoses, through an examination for herpes zoster, if vesicles are present, clinicians need to check serum antibodies. It is also possible that ACE, HIV, and inflammatory indicators could be tested in certain clinical settings. Cerebrospinal fluid (CSF) is typically not helpful in the diagnosis for facial paralysis, but it can differentiate it from diseases involving the CNS.

9.7 Medical Management and Treatment of Facial Paralysis

A discussion on the most common cause of facial paralysis, Bell palsy, will be followed by a general overview of the correct management of the clinically significant symptoms.

9.7.1 Bell Palsy

Most patients presenting with Bell palsy are otherwise healthy and fully recover spontaneously within weeks.[48] Following the standard Cochrane methodology, a study in 2016 affirmed that corticosteroids such as prednisone (a potent anti-inflammatory agent) are thought to limit facial nerve damage by reducing inflammation and are thus recommended.[49] In line with the findings by the American Academy of Otolaryngology-Head and Neck Surgery Foundation, the Royal Australian College of General Practitioners recommends the following[50]:

- With patients aged 16 years and older, provision of oral corticosteroids should occur 72 hours after symptom onset. However, the benefits of administration post 72 hours are unclear.[50,51,52]
- Recommended dosages are listed in ▶ Table 9.1

Noted in ▶ Table 9.1, historically, antivirals have also been prescribed in combination with corticosteroids to patients. Presently, guidelines recommend either the provision in combination with corticosteroids within 72 hours of symptom onset or for management of patients who present with vesicular rashes which is suggestive of viral infections such as HSV.[4]

Patients who are suffering from Bell palsy encounter paralysis of the orbicularis oculi muscle and may not be able to close their eyes fully.[50] This leads to an increased risk of foreign objects entering and potentially, affecting the ocular structures. As per the RACGP recommended management: educate patients to

Table 9.1 Various medical management techniques for the different causative factors of facial paralysis

Types of facial paralysis	Medical management
Bell palsy	Prednisone (anti-inflammatory agent) 1 mg/kg PO or 60 mg/d for 5 d then tapered over 5 d, for a total of 10 d[51] Antiviral therapy[a]: acyclovir (400 mg five times daily) and valacyclovir (1,000 mg three times daily).[51]
Herpes zoster virus	Famciclovir[b] (250 mg three times a day for 7 d, or if immunocompromised 500 mg three times a day for 10 d) and valacyclovir (1 g three times a day for 7 d).[51] Intravenous acyclovir (10 mg/kg three times a day) is usually reserved for immunocompromised patients with disseminated disease.[51] Cautious prescription for adverse effects of high-dose valacyclovir in VZV, with patients on corticosteroid, pregnant, or with an active infection or immunocompromised[51]
Herpes simplex virus reactivation	Recurrence: episodic therapy—valacyclovir 500 mg PO, BD for 3 d, famciclovir 1 g PO, BD for 1 d[51] Recurrence: suppressive therapy—valacyclovir 500 mg PO, daily for 6 mo, famciclovir 250 mg PO, BD for 6 mo[51]
Lyme disease	Although Lyme disease does not exist in Australia and as such no management protocols have been developed, the American national health body (CDC) has recommended antibiotic therapy for a few weeks such as doxycycline against *Borrelia burgdorferi* with the majority of patients usually recovering from both acute and chronic Lyme disease[51]
Acute otitis media	Antibiotic therapy with or without corticosteroids. Myringotomy (small incision in the eardrum) is also advised.[53]
Chronic suppurative otitis media	Antibiotics are indicated in all cases. Depending on the pathogenesis, surgical intervention may be indicated: myringotomy, mastoidectomy, nerve decompression, excision of a cholesteatoma[53]
Parotid neoplasm	For benign neoplasm, treatment primarily aimed at surgical removal of the neoplastic mass and subsequent symptom management of reduced stimulated salivation due to loss of one side of the parotid as per recommendations under **Sensory Trunk** in medical management.[54] For malignant parotid neoplasm, it is usually as a result of distant metastasis spread; so, management involves both surgical removal and adjunctive radiotherapy.[54] Due to the radiotherapy for metastatic management, all salivary glands are affected and patients are advised to not only follow the recommendations made under **Sensory Trunk** in medical management but may also consider salivary substitutes and atropine agonistic drugs such as Cevimeline provided there is residual salivary function[52]
Stroke	The majority of ischemic stroke patients will be treated by a combination of antithrombotic therapy, rehabilitation, and specific symptom management dependent on patient-specific presenting symptoms.[51] Caution is to be taken if antithrombotics are used and performing surgical procedures that may induce bleeding. Reference should be made to appropriate INR values in the therapeutic guidelines for procedures
Trauma	Primarily, there is surgical management according to their condition with appropriate symptom relief[55]
Genetic syndromes	Similar to trauma-induced facial paralysis, the management of genetic syndromes is symptom relief of facial paralysis[52]

[a]Clinical trial has shown that antiviral therapy in combination with corticosteroid therapy is of no additional benefit, compared with corticosteroid therapy alone.
[b]Famciclovir and valacyclovir are the preferred drugs given their greater bioavailability and less frequent dosing in comparison to acyclovir.

wear sunglasses when outdoors, use eye lubrication products such as muscarinic agonist eyedrops or their equivalent regularly as there is decreased lacrimation from paralysis of the lacrimal glands also, and tape the eyelid shut overnight when sleeping to prevent keratoconjunctivitis sicca and entrance of foreign objects.[50] Finally, patients are advised to consult with their family doctor if they experience any changes in vision, eye irritation, or pain.

With regard to adjunctive forms of treatment such as acupuncture, physiotherapy or electrotherapy, and surgical procedures, the RACGP currently has no recommendations due to a lack of both quality research and data.[50]

9.8 Symptoms Relief and Specific Intervention

9.8.1 Paralysis of Motor Trunk of Facial Nerve

Oral Dysfunctions

One of the clinically significant structures implicated is the orbicularis oris muscle.[3] Paralysis of the muscle prevents contraction of its fibers which slightly elevates and draws the lips together. Therefore, oral manifestations of facial paralysis are related to an inability to contain food, resting salivary production, and difficulty in normal speech production as the lips cannot purse to pronounce letters like "o."[1] Management involves educating the patient to eat slower and have smaller bites to reduce the amount of food that needs to be held in the mouth at any one time and therefore, the amount of contraction required by the orbicularis oris muscle to contain the food.[56] Indirectly, smaller portions of food will also aid with swallowing as there is more saliva relative to food to form the bolus. Finally, a slight upward tilt of the head will help prevent saliva drooling and pooling toward the buccal aspect which can lead to other medical implications such as angular cheilitis.[56]

Many of the superficial muscles of facial expression converge to insert on a vertical musculotendinous raphe lateral to the corner of the mouth known as the Modiolus.[1] Loss of this muscle tonicity in facial paralysis will lead to unsupported tissue drooping over the corner of the mouth, further compounding the symptoms of drooling and difficulty with normal speech. Simply supporting the paralyzed corner of the lip with a finger can greatly aid with day-to-day quality of life.

Paralysis of posterior belly of the digastric muscle inhibits the contraction of the muscle and in turn, prevents elevation of the hyoid bone which is involved in the depression of the mandible allowing for speech and the oral stage of swallowing.[1] Note that in conditions of facial nerve palsy only, the laryngeal and pharyngeal phases of swallowing are unaffected as those structures are innervated by other cranial nerves.[56] Likewise, paralysis of the stylohyoid muscle prevents the backward draw of the hyoid bone and elevation of the tongue, which is also involved in the oral stage of swallowing and speech. Correct management of dysphagia and difficulty with speech and language in addition to the medical intervention for each etiology outlined above includes transitioning to a softer, pureed diet or in severe cases, use of feeding tubes.[56]

Stapedius Muscle

The stapedius muscle dampens the vibrations of the stapes, regulating the amplitude of the sound waves generated and transmits it to the auditory ossicles.[1] Paralysis of the stapedius reduces this dampening, resulting in an increased amplitude of sound wave generated. This leads to a heightened response of the auditory ossicles known as hyperacusis. Treatment is commonly retraining therapy where patients slowly rebuild their tolerance to sounds.[52]

9.8.2 Sensory Trunk

Taste disturbances to the anterior two-thirds of the tongue and the palate are not clinically significant as patients with unilateral paralysis can still perceive taste through other taste receptors throughout the oral cavity.[51] Of greater clinical significance is the paralysis of parasympathomimetic secretomotor fibers of the sensory trunk innervating the submandibular salivary gland, sublingual salivary gland, and lacrimal glands. As mentioned in the prevention of corneal damage in Bell palsy, the same techniques can be extended to manage decreased lacrimation from facial paralysis of all causes.[52]

The submandibular and sublingual salivary glands account for the majority of resting salivary secretions.[3] Reduced salivation not only places the patients at increased risk of xerostomia and dental diseases such as caries or periodontal diseases from reduced salivary buffering but also at increased difficulty with chewing and swallowing due to reduced saliva to form the bolus. As outlined in the Australian Therapeutic guidelines, the following recommendations should be made to the patient for management of decreased salivation[51,52]:

- Ensure adequate hydration: drink adequate amounts of water, particularly fluoridated tap water which will also assist with remineralization of dental tissues.
- Consumption of noncariogenic, non-milk-extrinsic sugar, chewy foods that will stimulate salivary flow. Furthermore, as there is reduced salivary secretion from facial paralysis, the patient should chew thoroughly prior to swallowing so that there is enough saliva to form the bolus and the food particles are smaller from the prolonged masticatory cycling that aids digestion.
- Limit caffeine, alcohol, and tobacco use as these products reduce salivation that would further exaggerate the patient's symptoms.
- Patients should avoid alcohol-containing mouthwashes as there is a very high risk of dental erosion due to a lack of saliva flow and, in turn, buffering capacity. If patients are indicated for a mouthwash, patients should use a bicarbonate mouthwash instead that is nonacidic.
- From a dietary perspective, patients should limit cariogenic food intakes such as fermentable carbohydrates, as the decreased salivation lowers the ability of saliva to protect the dental hard tissues by buffering acids generated by micro-organism metabolism of these food sources.

9.9 Management of a Dental Patient with Facial Paralysis

Patients suffering from facial paralysis (FP) often present with muscle weakness, and this can affect their ability to carry out daily tasks of eating, drinking, talking, and smiling. Over time, these place a barrier to dental care that make it harder to maintain oral health. It is therefore important for dentists to recognize and understand its associated difficulties so that they can appropriately manage their patients.

9.9.1 Local Anesthetic

With local anesthetic integral to many dental procedures, temporary facial paralysis may occur following a misdirected inferior alveolar nerve block. If symptoms are observed, the practitioner should cease treatment and undergo an evaluation.[52] This includes checking for mouth-and-eye control by asking the patient to blink and smile. The patient should be monitored until some blinking returns and escorted home to remove the need for the patient to drive. It is important to note, however, that FP may sometimes not manifest for some time after treatment and, as a result, may develop after a patient has left the dental office.[33] In all cases, dentists should follow up on patients to check if any problems have occurred.

9.9.2 Restorative Treatment

All dental work aims to improve the quality of life of patients and so it is important to consider the benefits of treatment and weigh them against the cons. Often for individuals affected by FP, extensive work is simply not possible; however, for treatment that is available, the patient's comfort, dignity, and autonomy should be prioritized.[57] Indeed, the muscle-impairing nature of FP means that patients will usually find it difficult to open their mouth and maintain it for the length of treatment. To assist with this, bite blocks may be used to eliminate the need to manually open mouths, as well as dental rubber dams to prevent saliva and fluid contamination of the pulp. Treatment times can be more spread out than normal and multiple appointments can be arranged so that the patient is comfortable and receives the best outcome. In light of reduced salivary flow associated with the condition, there is likely an increased risk of dental caries and periodontal disease due to the absence of a buffer and natural antimicrobial.[57] For this reason, the preferred restorative materials should be the fluoride-releasing glass ionomer cement (GIC) to help with remineralization of enamel or the longer lasting, more durable amalgam.[57]

9.9.3 Root Caries

The prominence of root caries and neurological conditions increases with age. It is unsurprising then that facial paralysis is linked with the two, and this is evidenced by a 2010 survey that recorded a rate of 39% in the institutionalized elderly.[57] Treatment of root caries is, however, difficult due to the lack of access and should be delayed until FP resolves or is proven to be absolutely necessary. Instead, remedies should be focused on plaque control through mouthwashes, gels, or varnish as well as topical fluoride application to arrest present decay.[52] All of these can be delivered in higher concentrations by a dentist. Sometimes, in more exposed roots, the affected surface can be made more amenable to preventive measures through the action of a rotary instrument. This involves a smoothing out of the pupal floor and may or may not involve GIC placement.[57]

9.9.4 Extractions

Primary concerns surrounding dental extractions revolve around whether a patient will bleed excessively during treatment and their ability to form blood clots postoperatively. An understanding of antiplatelet and oral anticoagulants is thus required as these medications are common in the treatment of FP.[16] Current findings indicate aspirin and warfarin do not need to be discontinued prior to treatment, given that the patient's recent international normalized ratio (INR) is less than 4.0.[57] To

help with recovery, sutures and absorbable hemostatic material can be applied to the tooth socket(s).

9.9.5 Prosthodontics

All prosthodontic devices require careful consideration as they demand the removal of nonreplaceable, natural teeth. Moreover, a certain criterion such as a good level of oral stability must be met so that the denture can adapt to the mouth for proper use. These factors can present as an issue for FP patients, whose lowered degree of muscular control means that there are potential problems in adjusting to the new prosthesis.[57] In such case, a copy technique may be employed to create a custom denture with an improved fit surface. An additional issue faced by FP patients is the inability for sulcus elimination on their affected side. This results in a build-up of food debris on the buccal surface of the lower denture, creating an environment where cariogenic bacteria can flourish.[16,57] Management of this involves placement of an acrylic resin material on the denture surface or by moving the device more buccally to remove the space where food may accumulate.

9.9.6 Prior to and during Dental Procedure

An oral health practitioner can encounter a dental patient with a facial paralysis, be the first one to diagnose a patient with facial paralysis or induce facial paralysis iatrogenically during simple or complex dental procedures. Facial paralysis can negatively impact on a patient's oral health status as well as physical and emotional status. Therefore, an oral health practitioner should be able to diagnose a patient by clinical examination which can lead to early intervention and the treatment of the condition. Taking a good note of the medical history and medication is of great importance prior to the treatment. Also, a sound knowledge of facial anatomy and precautions during dental treatment for the high-risk patients are required for prevention of iatrogenic facial paralysis.

Patients with facial paralysis tend to show compromised oral function; hence, they can be considered to be high caries–risk patients. They often experience low salivary clearance level, low buffering capacity, food retention, and decreased oral vestibular cleansing capacity that lead to increased risk in developing oral diseases.[58] Use of fluoride mouthwash, saliva substitute products, and electric antioscillation toothbrush can be recommended to aid such patients in the maintenance of oral hygiene level. Prior to the dental procedure, an oral health practitioner should use the algorithm of questions shown in ▶ Fig. 9.4 in order to gain sufficient information before proceeding to treatment.[59] In case of the central facial paralysis caused by a stroke, a patient may be under anticoagulant or antiplatelet that interferes with blood clotting after invasive dental operation.[59] Communication with GP or hematologist is required

to adjust the dosage of the medications for the patients prior to dental treatment. During dental treatment, use of prop can be offered to maintain mouth opening for visualization and access into the oral cavity. In addition, rubber dam must be used for a good isolation and prevention of ingestion or inhalation of any debris from handpiece operation or small dental equipment. This is due to patient's decreased gag reflex that increases the chance of inhalation.[60]

Incident rates of facial paralysis after dental manipulation are much lower when compared to the other causes, and the incident rate can be further reduced by oral health practitioners if they take certain precautions.[61] Iatrogenic facial paralysis can be categorized into immediate or delayed.[62] The latter is often more severe than the former and takes longer to recover from.[63] Local anesthetics (LA) are believed to be the most responsible agent for

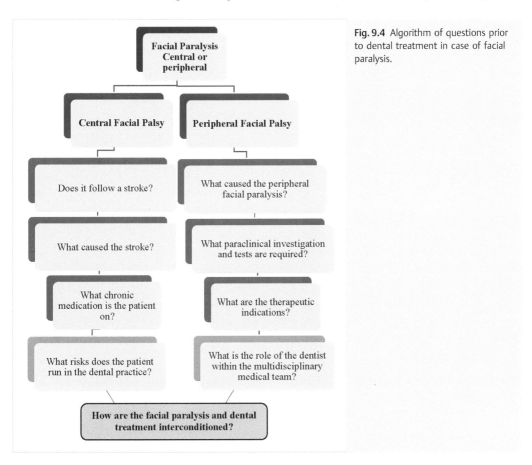

Fig. 9.4 Algorithm of questions prior to dental treatment in case of facial paralysis.

iatrogenic facial paralysis.[61] The most feasible mechanisms of LA include ischemic damage to the facial nerve caused by sympathetic vascular reflex, toxicity, mechanical effect of needle, and reactivation of herpes simplex virus or varicella zoster virus.[61,62] It is argued that reactivation of dormant viruses can also be triggered by stress, fear, hyperextension of the jaw, rough dental manipulation, prolonged use of dental equipment such as handpieces, prongs, and triplex syringe. There are rare cases where direct nerve damage occurs during osteotomy.[61,64] Prior to the dental procedure, an oral health practitioner must identify whether a patient has previous experience with HSV or HZV infection which increases the chance of developing iatrogenic facial paralysis.[64] They must be informed that there is a chance of developing facial paralysis that can be transient or prolonged before proceeding to dental treatment.[64] If the patient is currently showing symptoms of HSV or HZV, then the treatment must be postponed until existing symptoms disappear. Both a patient with the previous history of HSV or HZV and a patient with current symptoms of HSV or HZV should use prophylactic medication such as acyclovir, prednisone to reduce the chance of developing virus-responsible facial paralysis after dental manipulation.[61,64] During dental procedures, it is critical to know facial anatomy when administering LA and the use of correct dosage to prevent toxicity. Allowing a break during a long procedure reduces stress and stretching on muscle and nerve. Recommendation of anxiolytic drugs is an option to reduce mental stress. Avoid prolonged air blow into the socket after tooth extraction.[64]

9.10 Oral Medicine Aspects of Facial Paralysis

The oral cavity and associated structures suffer as a result of facial paralysis either due to direct symptoms of facial paralysis, or indirectly due to the patient having difficulty maintaining proper oral care and hygiene.

9.10.1 Xerostomia-related Issues

Due to the facial nerve supplying the sublingual and submandibular salivary glands, patients may experience xerostomia or a decrease in resting saliva secretion into the oral cavity. As saliva plays several critical roles in the oral cavity, the risk and prevalence of other oral pathologies and issues increases.[65] Risk of caries development would rise due to the absence of saliva to sufficiently neutralize the acids produced by bacteria as well as the inability to help flush away food debris and remineralize enamel.

Xerostomia also predisposes the patient to higher risks of oral fungal infections, notably candidiasis. It has been found that salivary flow is inversely related to the number of *Candida* species, and thus patients with xerostomia will experience higher levels of *Candida* species in the oral cavity.[66]

Burning mouth syndrome (BMS) is a painful condition that affects the oral mucosa of the mouth, which presents itself as a burning or tingling pain. BMS is characterized as primary or secondary, where primary BMS does not result from an underlying medical condition and secondary BMS results from an underlying medical condition.[67] Although not definitively determined yet, links between xerostomia and BMS have been noted, in which saliva and its flow rate may play an important role in both the initiation and maintenance of secondary BMS.[68,69]

9.10.2 Hygiene-related Oral Issues

In the vestibule of the paralyzed side of the oral cavity, there will be food accumulation and it may result in the build-up of plaque on the surfaces of teeth due to decrease in masticatory and facial muscle function. Therefore, this may result in an increased risk of periodontal diseases such as gingivitis and periodontitis, as well as dental decay. To further this problem, patients may have trouble maintaining proper oral hygiene due to difficulty opening their mouth and accessing certain parts of their mouth when either brushing or flossing on the affected side. Chemical plaque control through mouth-rinses is also compromised due to loss of function of facial muscles which are required for swishing the fluid around the oral cavity, and even retaining the liquid in the mouth may prove difficult due to a decrease in the muscular force of the lips.[70,71] It is therefore indicated that the patient makes regular appointments with a dental practitioner to ensure oral health is maintained.

9.10.3 Angular Cheilitis

The loss of motor function of the facial muscles, such as the orbicularis oris, also poses other problems around the oral cavity. On the paralyzed side, the oral commissure will droop and lead to the accumulation of saliva at the commissure of the mouth. Furthermore, the lip force and lip sealing ability of patient will be significantly reduced, which can result in further leakage of saliva from the mouth during mastication and difficulty in the retention of liquids during drinking. This can then result in angular cheilitis due to an infection by *Candida albicans*, *Staphylococcus aureus*, and B-hemolytic streptococci resulting in a cracking and possible ulceration at the corner of the mouth.[72] Antifungals and antibiotics are indicated in the treatment of angular cheilitis should it occur.

9.10.4 Temporomandibular Joint Issues

In a study on the relationship between facial paralysis and lateral preference in mastication, it is noted that about 70% of patients suffering from peripheral facial paralysis preferred to chew on the unaffected side of the mouth. Furthermore, a significant difference in size between the buccinator on the paralyzed side and unaffected side could be seen, possibly indicating reliance on their unaffected side for chewing.[73] Since the facial nerve innervates the buccinator muscle through the buccal branch, patients with facial palsy may find it difficult to chew effectively on the affected side. The buccinator is an accessory muscle of mastication that functions to push the cheek

against the teeth and keep the food bolus between the occluding surfaces of the teeth and thus plays an important role in the mastication process. Studies on unilateral chewing show that having a preferential side of chewing may cause temporomandibular joint (TMJ) issues and present with more symptoms of temporomandibular-related disorders (TMD) on the corresponding side.[74,75] Therefore, a patient suffering from unilateral facial palsy may be more prone to the development of signs and symptoms of TMD due to their preferred lateral chewing.

9.11 Coordination of Care between Dentist and Physician

Careful communication between dentists and medical practitioners is needed when treating patients who may be on anticoagulants such as warfarin, with careful monitoring of their INR. If the INR score is above 4, any dental surgery is contraindicated and must be referred to the medical practitioner.[52] It is also important for the dentist to take care when prescribing certain antibiotics or medications that could interact and alter the action of warfarin and interfere with the INR scores of the patient such as metronidazole.[76] In these cases, the dentist should communicate with the medical practitioner in charge of the patient's warfarin therapy.

As mentioned before, iatrogenic facial paralysis in the dental environment can be either caused by sympathetic vascular reflex, toxicity, mechanical effect of a needle, or through the secondary infections as a result of the injection such as HSV-1 or reactivation of the varicella zoster virus that can cause a delayed facial paralysis. It is therefore important to involve the medical practitioner and relevant medical specialties in determining and confirming the specific cause and etiology of the facial paralysis as it may be multifactorial and require treatment from other disciplines in order to provide the best possible outcome for the patient.[59]

As new etiological factors are being discovered, we are able to diagnose, treat, and manage the condition more effectively. Dentists should be aware of the impacts facial paralysis can have on their patients and how to manage the condition to improve the quality of patient's life.

References

[1] Baker EW, Schuenke M. Head and Neck Anatomy for Dental Medicine. New York: Thieme; 2010

[2] Kosins AM, Hurvitz KA, Evans GRD, Wirth GA. Facial paralysis for the plastic surgeon. Can J Plast Surg. 2007; 15(2):77–82

[3] Batista, KT. Facial paralysis: epidemiological analysis in a rehabilitation hospital. Rev Bras Cir Plást. 2011; 26(4):591–595

[4] Das AK, Sabarigirish K, Kashyap RC. Facial nerve paralysis: a three year retrospective study. Indian J Otolaryngol Head Neck Surg. 2006; 58(3):225–228

[5] Lin J, Chen Y, Wen H, Yang Z, Zeng J. Weakness of eye closure with central facial paralysis after unilateral hemispheric stroke predicts a worse outcome. J Stroke Cerebrovasc Dis. 2017; 26(4):834–841

[6] Shelley BP. Historical perspectives of facial palsy: before and after Sir Charles Bell to facial emotional expression. Arch Med Health Sci. 2013; 1(1):85–88

[7] Sajadi MM, Sajadi M-RM, Tabatabaie SM. The history of facial palsy and spasm. Neurology. 2011; 77(2):174–178

[8] Tabatabaei SM, Kalantar Hormozi A, Asadi M. Razi's description and treatment of facial paralysis. Arch Iran Med. 2011; 14(1):73–75

[9] Pearce JMS. Early observations on facial palsy. J Hist Neurosci. 2015; 24(4):319–325

[10] van de Graaf RC, Nicolai JP. Bell's palsy before Bell: Cornelis Stalpart van der Wiel's observation of Bell's palsy in 1683. Otol Neurotol. 2005; 26(6):1235–123–8

[11] Bird TD. Nicolaus A. Friedreich's description of peripheral facial nerve paralysis in 1798. J Neurol Neurosurg Psychiatry. 1979; 42(1):56–58

[12] Kosins AM, Hurvitz KA, Evans GR, Wirth GA. Facial paralysis for the plastic surgeon. Can J Plast Surg. 2007; 15(2):77–82

[13] Silva IdS. Cancer Epidemiology: Principles and Methods. France: International Agency for Research on Cancer; 1999

[14] Lamina S, Hanif S. Pattern of facial palsy in a typical Nigerian specialist hospital. Afr Health Sci. 2012; 12(4):514–517

[15] Peitersen E. Bell's palsy: the spontaneous course of 2,500 peripheral facial nerve palsies of different etiologies. Acta Otolaryngol Suppl. 2002(549):4–30

[16] Roob G, Fazekas F, Hartung HP. Peripheral facial palsy: etiology, diagnosis and treatment. Eur Neurol. 1999; 41(1):3–9

[17] Tomás-Roca L, Pérez-Aytés A, Puelles L, Marín F. In silico identification of new candidate genes for hereditary congenital facial paresis. Int J Dev Neurosci. 2011; 29(4):451–460

[18] Prescott CA. Idiopathic facial nerve palsy (the effect of treatment with steroids). J Laryngol Otol. 1988; 102(5):403–407

[19] Lorch M, Teach SJ. Facial nerve palsy: etiology and approach to diagnosis and treatment. Pediatr Emerg Care. 2010; 26(10):763–769, quiz 770–773

[20] Adour KK. Current concepts in neurology: diagnosis and management of facial paralysis. N Engl J Med. 1982; 307(6):348–351

[21] Kennedy PG. Key issues in varicella-zoster virus latency. J Neurovirol. 2002; 8 Suppl 2:80–84

[22] Sweeney CJ, Gilden DH. Ramsay Hunt syndrome. J Neurol Neurosurg Psychiatry. 2001; 71(2):149–154

[23] Murakami S, Mizobuchi M, Nakashiro Y, Doi T, Hato N, Yanagihara N. Bell palsy and herpes simplex virus: identification of viral DNA in endoneurial fluid and muscle. Ann Intern Med. 1996; 124(1)(, Pt 1):27–30

[24] McCormick DP. Herpes-simplex virus as a cause of Bell's palsy. Lancet. 1972; 1(7757):937–939

[25] Reik L, Steere AC, Bartenhagen NH, Shope RE, Malawista SE. Neurologic abnormalities of Lyme disease. Medicine (Baltimore). 1979; 58(4):281–294

[26] Joseph EM, Sperling NM. Facial nerve paralysis in acute otitis media: cause and management revisited. Otolaryngol Head Neck Surg. 1998; 118(5):694–696

[27] Yonamine FK, Tuma J, Silva RF, Soares MC, Testa JR. Facial paralysis associated with acute otitis media. Rev Bras Otorrinolaringol (Engl Ed). 2009; 75(2):228–230

[28] Savić DL, Djerić DR. Facial paralysis in chronic suppurative otitis media. Clin Otolaryngol Allied Sci. 1989; 14(6):515–517

[29] Dirnagl U, Iadecola C, Moskowitz MA. Pathobiology of ischaemic stroke: an integrated view. Trends Neurosci. 1999; 22(9):391–397

[30] Testai FD, Aiyagari V. Acute hemorrhagic stroke pathophysiology and medical interventions: blood pressure control, management of anticoagulant-associated brain hemorrhage and general management principles. Neurol Clin. 2008; 26(4):963–985, viii–ix

[31] Eneroth CM. Facial nerve paralysis. A criterion of malignancy in parotid tumors. Arch Otolaryngol. 1972; 95(4):300–304

[32] Jackson CG, Glasscock ME, III, Hughes G, Sismanis A. Facial paralysis of neoplastic origin: diagnosis and management. Laryngoscope. 1980; 90(10)(, Pt 1):1581–1595

[33] Gray RL. Peripheral facial nerve paralysis of dental origin. Br J Oral Surg. 1978; 16(2):143–150

[34] Crean SJ, Powis A. Neurological complications of local anaesthetics in dentistry. Dent Update. 1999; 26(8):344–349

[35] Steinfeldt T, Nimphius W, Werner T, et al. Nerve injury by needle nerve perforation in regional anaesthesia: does size matter? Br J Anaesth. 2010; 104(2):245–253

[36] Kadakia S, Helman SN, Schwedhelm T, Saman M, Azizzadeh B. Examining the genetics of congenital facial paralysis–a closer look at Moebius syndrome. Oral Maxillofac Surg. 2015; 19(2):109–116

[37] Gutowski NJ, Chilton JK. The congenital cranial dysinnervation disorders. Arch Dis Child. 2015; 100(7):678–681

[38] Tomas-Roca L, Tsaalbi-Shtylik A, Jansen JG, et al. De novo mutations in PLXND1 and REV3 L cause Möbius syndrome. Nat Commun. 2015; 6:7199

[39] Berker N, Acaroğlu G, Soykan E. Goldenhar's syndrome (oculo-auriculo-vertebral dysplasia) with congenital facial nerve palsy. Yonsei Med J. 2004; 45(1):157–160

[40] Cleiren E, Bénichou O, Van Hul E, et al. Albers-Schönberg disease (autosomal dominant osteopetrosis, type II) results from mutations in the ClCN7 chloride channel gene. Hum Mol Genet. 2001; 10(25):2861–2867

[41] Kulkarni GB, Pal PK, Shyambabu C, Kovoor JME, Senthilkumar E. Osteopetrosis manifesting as recurrent bilateral facial palsy in childhood: a case report. Clin Neurol Neurosurg. 2011; 113(3):230–234

[42] Liu R, Yu S. Melkersson-Rosenthal syndrome: a review of seven patients. J Clin Neurosci. 2013; 20(7):993–995

[43] Sun B, Zhou C, Han Z. Facial palsy in Melkersson-Rosenthal syndrome and Bell's palsy: familial history and recurrence tendency. Ann Otol Rhinol Laryngol. 2015; 124(2):107–109

[44] Uyguner ZO, Toksoy G, Altunoglu U, Ozgur H, Basaran S, Kayserili H. A new hereditary congenital facial palsy case supports arg5 in HOX-DNA binding domain as possible hot spot for mutations. Eur J Med Genet. 2015; 58(6–7): 358–363

[45] Somasundara D, Sullivan F. Management of Bell's palsy. Aust Prescr. 2017; 40(3):94–97

[46] Phillips KM, Heiser A, Gaudin R, Hadlock TA, Jowett N. Onset of Bell's palsy in late pregnancy and early puerperium is associated with worse long-term outcomes. Laryngoscope. 2017; 127(12):2854–2859

[47] Cooper L, Branagan-Harris M, Tuson R, Nduka C. Lyme disease and Bell's palsy: an epidemiological study of diagnosis and risk in England. Br J Gen Pract. 2017; 67(658):e329–e335

[48] McCaul JA, Cascarini L, Godden D, Coombes D, Brennan PA, Kerawala CJ. Evidence based management of Bell's palsy. Br J Oral Maxillofac Surg. 2014; 52(5):387–391

[49] de Almeida JR, Jr, Guyatt GH, Sud S, et al. Bell Palsy Working Group, Canadian Society of Otolaryngology - Head and Neck Surgery and Canadian Neurological Sciences Federation. Management of Bell palsy: clinical practice guideline. CMAJ. 2014; 186(12):917–922

[50] Phan NT, Panizza B, Wallwork B. A general practice approach to Bell's palsy. Aust Fam Physician. 2016; 45(11):794–797

[51] Pasha R. Otolaryngology Head and Neck Surgery: Clinical Reference Guide. Plural Publishing: 2017

[52] Therapeutic Guidelines. Oral and Dental. Melbourne, Australia: Therapeutic Guidelines Limited; 2012

[53] Acuin J. Chronic suppurative otitis media. Clin Evid. 2004 (12):710–729

[54] Bussu F, Parrilla C, Rizzo D, Almadori G, Paludetti G, Galli J. Clinical approach and treatment of benign and malignant parotid masses, personal experience. Acta Otorhinolaryngol Ital. 2011; 31(3):135–143

[55] Gordin E, Lee TS, Ducic Y, Arnaoutakis D. Facial nerve trauma: evaluation and considerations in management. Craniomaxillofac Trauma Reconstr. 2015; 8(1):1–13

[56] Wax MK. Facial Paralysis: A Comprehensive Rehabilitative Approach. 1st ed. San Diego, CA: Plural Publishing Inc; 2017

[57] Guidelines for Oral Healthcare for Stroke Survivors: British Society of Gerodontology; 2010. Available at: https://www.gerodontology.com/content/uploads/2014/10/stroke_guidelines.pdf. Accessed May 15, 2019

[58] Kato Y, Kamo H, Kobayashi A, et al. Quantitative evaluation of oral function in acute and recovery phase of idiopathic facial palsy; a preliminary controlled study. Clin Otolaryngol. 2013; 38(3):231–236

[59] Ilea A, Cristea A, Tărmure V, Trombitaş VE, Câmpian RS, Albu S. Management of patients with facial paralysis in the dental office: a brief review of the literature and case report. Quintessence Int. 2014; 45(1):75–86

[60] Frost L. Dental management of the tropical disease human African trypanosomiasis: an unusual case of pseudobulbar palsy. Br Dent J. 2011; 210(1):13–16

[61] Gaudin RA, Remenschneider AK, Phillips K, et al. Facial palsy after dental procedures - Is viral reactivation responsible? J Craniomaxillofac Surg. 2017; 45(1):71–75

[62] Misirlioglu M, Adisen M, Okkesim A, Akyil Y. Facial nerve paralysis after dental procedure. Journal of Oral and Maxillofacial Radiology.. 2016; 4(3):80–82

[63] Tzermpos FH. Transient delayed facial nerve palsy after inferior alveolar nerve block anesthesia. Anesth Prog. 2012; 59 (1):22–27

[64] Madhulaxmi NV, Wahab A. Facial nerve palsy in dental procedures – a review article. Int J Clin Dentistry. 2015; 8(3): 263–270

[65] Villa A, Connell CL, Abati S. Diagnosis and management of xerostomia and hyposalivation. Ther Clin Risk Manag. 2014; 11:45–51

[66] Shinozaki S, Moriyama M, Hayashida JN, et al. Close association between oral Candida species and oral mucosal disorders in patients with xerostomia. Oral Dis. 2012; 18(7):667–672

[67] National Institute of Dental and Craniofacial Research. Burning Mouth Syndrome: National Institutes of Health; 2016. Available at: https://www.nidcr.nih.gov/OralHealth/Topics/Burning/BurningMouthSyndrome.htm. Accessed May 15, 2019

[68] Chimenos-Kustner E, Marques-Soares MS. Burning mouth and saliva. Med Oral. 2002; 7(4):244–253

[69] Lee YC, Hong IK, Na SY, Eun YG. Evaluation of salivary function in patients with burning mouth syndrome. Oral Dis. 2015; 21(3):308–313

[70] Klobucar R, Kingsmill V, Venables V, Bisase B, Nduka C. A dental perspective of facial palsy. Faculty Dental Journal.. 2012; 3(4):202–207

[71] Schimmel M, Leemann B, Herrmann FR, Kiliaridis S, Schnider A, Müller F. Masticatory function and bite force in stroke patients. J Dent Res. 2011; 90(2):230–234

[72] Devani A, Barankin B. Answer: can you identify this condition? Can Fam Physician. 2007; 53(6):1022–1023

[73] Rahal A, Goffi-Gomez MV. Clinical and electromyographic study of lateral preference in mastication in patients with longstanding peripheral facial paralysis. Int J Orofacial Myology. 2009; 35:19–32

[74] Reinhardt R, Tremel T, Wehrbein H, Reinhardt W. The unilateral chewing phenomenon, occlusion, and TMD. Cranio. 2006; 24(3):166–170

[75] Tiwari S, Nambiar S, Unnikrishnan B. Chewing side preference - Impact on facial symmetry, dentition and temporomandibular joint and its correlation with handedness. J Orofac Sci. 2017; 9(1):22–27

[76] Woods RG, Savage N. Managing dental patients receiving warfarin therapy. Aust Prescr. 2002; 25:69

Index

Note: Page numbers set **bold** or *italic* indicate headings or figures, respectively.